Simple
fitter, happier, stronger you

Let's Walk Nordic

Vicky Welsh

Rethink

Disclaimer:
The use of any information in this book, including any suggested exercise, is solely at the reader's own risk. You should always seek medical advice before undertaking any exercise or starting an exercise programme. Neither Rethink Press nor the author can be held liable or responsible in respect of any and all injuries, losses, damages, expense, or other adverse effects incurred while undertaking any of the exercise or other activities described in this book.

For Adrian

and

for Chris, Matt and Sammy

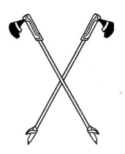

CONTENTS

FOREWORD

As a doctor specialising for many years in healthy weight loss, I know the immense value of this book. I know that there is a lot more to exercise than burning calories, though many of us trying to lose weight will focus on that alone. Then exercise becomes yet another demand on our time, adding to our list of things we should do…or making us feel guilty if we don't.

When I first met Vicky, many years ago, I knew she understood that exercise holds so much more value than that. I wasn't familiar with Nordic walking at that time, but thanks to Vicky's passion and in-depth understanding, I discovered that Nordic walking provides all of the amazing benefits that the best forms of exercise can bring. It's sociable and fun – great for boosting hormones that help mental health. It builds muscle – a vital and often under-valued factor in health and weight loss. It strengthens bones and helps stabilise joints by improving proprioception. It gets you outdoors for fresh air and natural light which re-set the body clock and sleep cycle, helping health and weight-control too. It improves posture and core-stability, reducing the risk of injury and easing pain. And exercise also helps reduce insulin resistance – one of the factors associated with the diseases that many of us suffer from now.

I could go on, but if you aren't yet familiar with Nordic walking, just try it! With Vicky's expert guidance and enthusiasm, you'll soon know how much happier your body and mind will feel. And for those already familiar with Nordic walking, the expert tips in this book will help you take your exercise safely to a new level – whether you are trying to lose weight, tackle specific health issues or simply to have fun and keep fit in a way that you can continue for many years to come.

Dr Sally Norton, MBChB MD FRCS, www.drsallynorton.com

INTRODUCTION

It is so important that we are physically active but lots of us struggle to find an activity that is effective and which we enjoy. It's easy to get caught up in thinking you need to go to the gym or do something exceptional to improve your health, fitness and mental wellbeing. This is not the case.

As many of us discovered during the Covid-19 pandemic, walking connects you to nature, eases stress and anxiety, helps you tone up and lose weight, is a gateway to discovering the world around you and, most importantly, is enjoyable. The quiet underdog of the fitness world reminded us that we don't need expensive memberships, the latest gadgets, or gruelling workouts to get healthy.

And what if I told you there was an enhanced way of walking that could take this everyday activity to the next level? A way to make walking more dynamic, hitting that sweet spot of a whole-body, high-cardio, low-impact exercise, while making it easier and more comfortable to walk if you have sore joints, back pain, or poor balance. Nordic walking is that activity and *Let's Walk Nordic* is a practical guide showing you how to Nordic walk and use it to improve your health and fitness.

I came across Nordic walking twelve years ago. I'd had an auto-immune disease in my mid-thirties that had caused a great deal of joint pain and put an end to my running days. I still had to be careful when exercising as my joints were vulnerable to flare-ups, so I was looking for a sustainable, holistic form of exercise that would get my heart rate up and keep me fit and healthy without hurting my joints. It also had to be something that

I could slot into my day, doubling up as a dog walk and social activity that I could enjoy with friends.

At the time, Nordic walking was relatively new to the UK, but my mother-in-law had joined a local group in Norfolk and suggested I try it out. As a personal trainer, I had heard of Nordic walking, but I thought it was for older people or those recovering from illness or injury. From my first session, I was blown away. I knew that Nordic walking was based on regular walking using two poles (my mistake of calling them 'sticks' was quickly corrected) to add support and engage your upper body. I had no idea, though, that it also teaches you correct posture and body alignment. It was like an outdoors walking Pilates experience, boosting balance and strength in a supportive, holistic way. It was energetic and lots of fun.

I could feel my back tension easing and my arms and upper body working, and I could go much faster than regular walking. The best thing was, to my utter delight, my joints didn't hurt. It felt easy and natural. Everyone was chatting and enjoying themselves, and even though we had different fitness levels we were all getting a good cardiovascular workout.

I fell in love with Nordic walking overnight and, at the same time, found a new career path. I stopped my gym-based personal training business and built a new one around Nordic walking, establishing an award-winning company that became one of the largest in the country. Since starting twelve years ago, I have taught over a thousand people to Nordic walk. They have spanned the entire fitness spectrum: people looking for something to help them lose weight, tone up and get fit; runners wanting an effective low-impact training option; people rehabilitating from hip or knee surgery; women going through the menopause seeking an effective means for weight loss and bone health but also something sociable; children wanting an alternative to mainstream sports; distance walkers wanting to improve their walking technique, speed and endurance; older clients who were becoming increasingly anxious about walking due to pain and balance worries; cancer patients Nordic walking through treatment; people with Parkinson's seeking a way to stay active and mobile. But above all, it was people with no particular purpose other than seeking a fun, sociable exercise that nurtured their mental wellbeing and kept them fit, healthy and active long into old age.

While Nordic walking is easy to learn, how much benefit you get from it depends on your technique. Nordic walking badly is not only a missed opportunity, but it can also perpetuate poor posture and walking habits. Driven by a desire to provide the best possible Nordic walking teaching, I have studied it from every angle, reading voraciously and having discussions with physios, chiropractors, podiatrists and biomechanical experts about how we use our muscles and how this knowledge can be overlayed onto Nordic walking to meet each person's unique needs. I have even been to Finland, the birthplace of Nordic walking, to see what I could glean about Nordic walking from Nordic skiing.

For years I have been sharing this information and knowledge through blogs, articles, talks and social media, attracting an international audience. With an increasing number of people wanting to Nordic walk and a lack of good books on the subject, I felt it was time to consolidate all my learning and experience and create the practical guide *Let's Walk Nordic*.

In Part One, I explain what Nordic walking is and compare it with running, regular walking and its closest cousin, trekking. I also explain the science behind why Nordic walking is such a powerful facilitator of health and fitness.

In Part Two, I set out the basic Nordic walking technique in a clear and simple way, giving you the Four Steps to Success. These are your foundations, from your posture and arm swing to your lower body action. In this section, you will pick up lots of handy tips for improving your regular walking too.

In Part Three, I discuss Nordic walking kit, walking intensity, goal setting and what warm-ups and stretches will support your Nordic walking health and fitness journey. In the final part of *Let's Walk Nordic*, I show you how to build on the foundations of Part Two and adapt your Nordic walking for your particular needs. There are menus to help you accommodate or perhaps resolve a bad back, tone up, reduce your stress, increase your walking confidence and much more.

Threaded throughout are walkers' stories about how Nordic walking has changed their lives, additional information and tips from health experts and links to videos and podcasts to help you on your Nordic walking journey.

Nordic walking is outdoors, sociable and non-competitive. You do not need to be good at sport to be good at Nordic walking (in fact, the people I've taught who have been best at it are generally those who hated sports at school). All you need are two poles and a knowledge of the correct technique. *Let's Walk Nordic* is your guide and gateway to a fitter, happier, stronger you.

PART ONE

WHAT IS NORDIC WALKING?

The first questions I'm usually asked about Nordic walking are: What is it? Where did it come from? And what does it have to offer? In this first part of the book, I answer these questions, giving a brief history of how Nordic walking came about and how it compares with regular walking, running and trekking. I also outline the science in support of the health and fitness benefits of Nordic walking.

ONE

Nordic Walking Explained

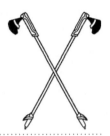

Nordic walking is a simple fitness activity which has its origins in cross-country skiing. It is a natural action based entirely on regular walking with the addition of two poles and a specific technique to turn your walk into a whole-body exercise. Nordic walking can be energetic, but if you are an inactive person or don't enjoy exercising, think of it as a supportive walk that uses all your main muscle groups, works your heart and lungs and improves your posture. It's easy to learn, effective, safe, fun and one of its great advantages, especially in this post Covid-19 world, is that it's an outdoors activity.

There are many things I like about Nordic walking, but right at the top of my list is adaptability. It's suitable for almost everyone, regardless of their age or physical condition, and it can improve health, increase fitness or be treated as a sport.

Given the immense health and fitness benefits of Nordic walking I still find it extraordinary that it only came into being as a fitness activity for all in the late 1990s and didn't arrive in the UK until the early 2000s. Elite cross-country skiers have been using their ski poles during the snowless off-season for decades to maintain their upper body strength and keep their fitness high, but it wasn't until Finnish health professionals recognised its potential for the general population that walking using poles 'cross-country skiing style' emerged.[1] The ski pole was shortened, a glove-type strap added and a technique for an enhanced walking style developed so that participants could walk in a biomechanically correct way and extend their range of arm swing for maximum benefit. The International Nordic Walking Federation (INWA) was formed in 2000 and rolled out an international education system to teach this new activity.

As Nordic walking was being established in Finland, Tom Rutlin was introducing a similar fitness activity in the USA.[2] Using his cross-country skiing and ski coaching knowledge, he developed strapless Exerstrider poles and a technique for using them that is similar to Nordic walking. It is still popular and widely used today.

Other organisations have since sprung up and developed their own style of Nordic walking. *Let's Walk Nordic* is based on the INWA technique.

Nordic walking versus regular walking

Many walkers are curious about what Nordic walking can offer over and above regular walking as a means of exercise. Walking is simple, it's in our DNA, but over the years most of us pick up sloppy walking habits without realising. Look around you and see how others walk: shoulders hunched, head dropped, arms hanging listlessly, hands in pockets, feet scuffing the ground and pointing in all directions except forward. Maybe you do some of these things yourself. A poor walking style perpetuates and exacerbates imbalances so if, for example, you have neck and shoulder tension, your current walking style will almost certainly be adding to it. If you don't use your feet properly you will most likely be heading for a fall – literally – in later years, as well as knee and back pain because you aren't using the right muscles in the right way.

The Nordic walking technique teaches correct posture for correct walking. It breaks the pattern of poor movement habits and trains your body to walk in a balanced way, including how to hold your skeleton (your spine, head, shoulders and chest in particular); how you use your arms; which muscles to engage, especially in your lower body; how to use your feet; and how to distribute your weight. Even if you're not interested in the activity of Nordic walking, there's lots from the technique that you can apply to your regular walking. Correct body movement learned while Nordic walking eventually spills over to your day-to-day walking, making your body better aligned and balanced with every step you take.

Nordic walking also uses more muscles than regular walking, which is one of its key benefits. The poles, coupled with the correct technique, engage your upper body and bring your arms, shoulders, chest, back and core stabilising muscles into the act of walking. Nordic walking strengthens and tones these areas, sculpting your arms, giving definition to your shoulders, working the pectoral muscles, which help firm your chest, and tightening your waist.

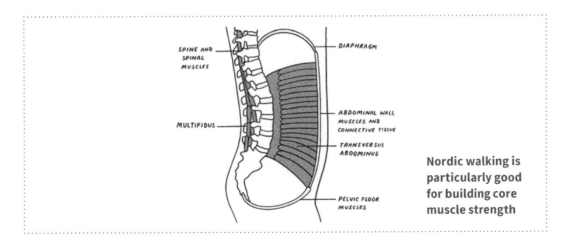

SPINE AND SPINAL MUSCLES

DIAPHRAGM

MULTIFIDUS

ABDOMINAL WALL MUSCLES AND CONNECTIVE TISSUE

TRANSVERSUS ABDOMINUS

PELVIC FLOOR MUSCLES

Nordic walking is particularly good for building core muscle strength

Your 'core' is the group of muscles that help protect your lower back, support your pelvis, legs and upper body, and improve your overall movement. It's often referred to as being like a pressurised container. The lid at the top is your diaphragm (your breathing muscle). Your deep abdominal muscles and your spinal muscles form the cylinder, and at the bottom sits your pelvic floor. All these muscles work in unison with each other and if any of them aren't working properly the container will start to lose pressure, weakening the stable base you need to move with ease and good balance.

The extra muscular demand that Nordic walking places on your body also makes it a great exercise for weight loss and weight management, if this is a health goal for you. It increases your heart rate and oxygen consumption and burns more calories than regular walking.[3] Despite this, Nordic walking feels easier than regular walking. The poles provide support, you're better aligned, which allows you to walk more freely, and the effort of walking is distributed between your upper and lower body.

Nordic walking's benefits over regular walking accelerate as you get older. I've already mentioned that it improves muscle tone and power. This becomes increasingly important as you age when muscles and balance begin to weaken. While walking is great for keeping your lower body strong, it does nothing for your upper body or your balance. Nordic walking, on the other hand, improves both – indeed, The UK Health Security Agency (UKHSA) – formerly Public Health England – specifically recommends it for muscle and balance strength. In their 2018 report, they rated Nordic walking higher than both walking and running for muscle and balance improvement.

Walking, despite cardiovascular and other health benefits, had a low beneficial effect on either bone health or falls reductions, with only small gains in muscle strength.

Other benefits of Nordic walking over regular walking include providing greater support and relieving joint and back pain, plus helping to maintain the range of motion of arms and shoulders. This means that simple everyday movements like reaching your arm back to put your coat on, twisting for your seatbelt in the car and doing zips or straps up at the back – all things that can become more difficult with age – continue to be straightforward.

Finally, Nordic walking is designed to propel you forward, which by nature increases your walking speed. If you struggle to keep up with friends and family, this is brilliant. No longer will they be striding out ahead while you valiantly try to keep up. This may seem a small point, but I've had many clients who wanted to learn Nordic walking specifically so they could match their partner's walking pace. It always worked and they sometimes even exceeded their partner's walking pace. Walking holidays became a pleasure for both parties; they protected their joints and increased their walking stamina while enjoying each other's company and the fresh air.

Comparison of running, walking, Nordic walking and cycling[4]

Type of sport, physical activity or exercise	Improvement in muscle function	Improvement in bone health	Improvement in balance
Running	x	xx	x
Walking	x	x	0
Nordic walking	xx	NK	xx
Cycling	x	x	x

Key: xxx = Strong effect; xx = medium; x = low; 0 = no effect; NK = not known
Taken from UKHSA (formerly Public Health England)

Nordic walking versus running

Running is a hugely popular exercise and for good reason – it's a natural body movement that strengthens your heart and lungs, burns lots of calories and is a great way of getting or staying fit and healthy. On top of that, it's time-efficient, social, fun and can be done anywhere. I'm a big fan of running and am certainly not about to try and persuade anyone to ditch it for Nordic walking. There are, however, some things to think about if you're a runner. The first is injuries.

Typically, 50% of runners injure themselves yearly.[5] Many factors are involved, of course, but by nature running is a high-impact exercise. This isn't a problem if you run with good technique and correct alignment, have built up gradually and aren't doing crazy distances. But if your running style is slightly off, you will be repeatedly landing your full body weight on a misaligned bodily structure with each stride. 'Runner's knee', shin splints and hip and lower back pain are all common and unwelcome companions for many runners. The more miles you run, the greater the risk of injury. Running is much less forgiving than walking, where you always have one foot on the ground.

If you're a runner reading this book, it might be because you've had enough injuries or niggles that you're considering Nordic walking as an alternative or as part of your rehab. It's worth noting that the biggest risk factor for a running injury is if you've previously been injured.

Nordic walking is a low-impact exercise that bridges the intensity divide between walking and running. While you can't go faster than you could running, Nordic walkers who are keen on speed can go quite fast and will frequently outstrip joggers going uphill. I've completed several half marathons with an average speed of 8km/h (5mph) and there are many Nordic walkers out there faster than me. It's a competitive activity in many countries, with an annual INWA World Cup for 21km and 10km distances. It's also possible to Nordic run and trail running poles are now commonly the same design as Nordic walking poles.

If you're repeatedly getting injured or running causes you pain, there's almost certainly an exercise out there that's better suited to you. For me, it was Nordic walking. As I said in the introduction, I had to give up running due to an auto-immune disease that affected my joints and made it too painful to run. It felt like a bereavement at the time but, as my story shows, there's light at the end of the tunnel. I have even been able to Nordic run without my joint problems recurring and have taught many Nordic walkers who are ex-runners.

If you love running but are aware of the injury risk and want to reduce the chances of that happening, Nordic walking can be used as a great cross-training tool, especially for endurance runners. It still provides a good aerobic workout but with lower impact. A study comparing Nordic walking and running at the same speeds (8km/h and 8.5km/h) found that the force exerted on the lower body was 36% lower in Nordic walking than running.[6] Plus Nordic walking works your entire body in a holistic, biomechanically correct way ensuring that you're strengthening your body as a whole.

This brings me onto my next point: Nordic walking is a whole-body fitness activity, running isn't. Adding the poles engages the core stabilising muscles in your trunk and strengthens your arms, shoulders and upper body in a way that running can't. To achieve the benefits that Nordic walking offers, a runner would need to do additional exercises working their arms, core and back. If you're someone who doesn't enjoy running and is doing it as a means to an end, you can achieve that pert bottom, trim waistline and toned legs through Nordic walking instead and you will get many additional benefits, such as improved posture, breathing and walking gait, at the same time. In addition, you can still get that 'runner's high' from Nordic walking. The exhilaration I get after an energetic Nordic walk is right up there with those from my running days. There are many things in life we do because we need or ought to. Exercise shouldn't be one of them. Find something you enjoy, and you are more likely to keep going and build it into your life in a sustainable way.

At some point in all our lives, there comes a moment when we have to assess the exercise we're doing, whether it's sufficient and whether it's suitable for us long term. There are certainly runners in their 70s and 80s, but I would suggest they are the exception rather than the rule. Nordic walking can be done throughout your whole life, right to the last. The same cannot generally be said for running.

PIPPA'S STORY

A friend had first recommended Nordic walking to me, but I claimed I was far too young, it wasn't energetic enough, it was too slow and off-beat. Two years later, I had grown tired of my high-intensity gym classes, couldn't run thanks to an ongoing back injury, and needed something to give me back my 'schwing'. I also wanted to be more of an 'outdoor girl', to enjoy all weathers and set my daughters a positive example.

So when a Nordic walking class started up in the park near my home, I decided to give it a go. I loved it from the moment I started.

I can't believe how much my fitness has increased. I have gone back to a bit of running as the Nordic walking technique has had such a positive effect on my core support and because of that, my back injury is far less problematic. I am more toned, happier as my exercise is now outdoors and I just love walking in the rain. To top it all, I have a clearer mind, my mood is much more upbeat, and I love my new relationship with nature.

There is a new phrase in the house, 'going Nordic' – as in, 'Mum's going Nordic'. I love that. It's my equivalent to 'going AWOL' for that all-important hour or two for myself.

Nordic walking versus trekking

I'm often asked how Nordic walking is any different from trekking with poles, given that they are both a form of walking with sticks. There's undoubtedly a crossover between two, but there are key differences in the design of the poles and how they are intended to be used.

Nordic walking is primarily intended as a fitness activity, adding poles to regular walking to increase fitness, strengthen posture and provide a whole range of other health benefits. To that end, the poles are designed to be angled backwards so that you can continue to walk in a natural way with a full arm swing. The pole handles are smooth and slender with a glove-type strap attached to facilitate the specific Nordic walking technique, allowing you to slide your hand along the grip and let go of the handle entirely, pushing through the strap so that you can swing your arm far behind your body. This increases the health and fitness benefits. Even the paws for covering the tip of the pole when walking on tarmac and other hard surfaces are slanted to ensure the correct pole angle and arm swing can be maintained whatever the terrain.

In contrast, trekking poles have a chunky grip, often with finger grooves and a ledge at the bottom to rest your hand on; this encourages your hand into a fixed position while you walk. They also have an adjustable looped strap which, depending on how you use it, can offer support for your hand while walking as well as keeping the poles attached to your wrist, should you let go for any reason. There's no angled paw at the bottom, just a rounded stopper.

Using poles is a long-established way of supporting you on a long walk or trek and making it easier to traverse rocky ground and up and down hills. But there's no particular technique for this and trekking poles are not designed to strengthen your posture or provide any specific health benefits. If you look around you, you will see that many people only use one pole and those who use two poles generally place them in front and in an upright position. The grip design encourages this vertical plant, but it means that your elbows are always bent, mostly at a right angle, and it's impossible to swing your arm to a full extension and in a natural way. Consequently, you are walking with an inhibited upper body action and arm swing. Even if you did angle your trekking poles backwards to allow your arms to swing naturally, it's simply not possible to extend your arm behind your body because the loop strap doesn't allow you to maintain control of the pole if you let go of the grip. The obvious impact of using just one trekking pole is that your body is not supported in a balanced way, and you'll be working one side of your upper body harder than the other, which is likely to have a knock-on effect throughout your body.

While you can't Nordic walk effectively using trekking poles, you can trek with Nordic walking poles. Done correctly, this will greatly boost your walking style, provide extra propulsion and enable you to trek long distances with good posture. I love using my Nordic walking poles on long hikes and have been able to complete some seriously challenging walks without blisters or pain. Where there are particularly difficult rocky or downhill sections, I just unclip my straps so that I'm not attached to the pole.

Trekking poles have been around for decades and are well loved and highly regarded as a walking aid, even though they don't facilitate a natural walking pattern. As the popularity of Nordic walking and the understanding of what it has to offer has grown, I have noticed the design of trekking poles changing. They are becoming lighter and the grips more ergonomically shaped. Some trekking poles and most trail running poles now have the Nordic walking style strap. This is good news as it increases the versatility of trekking poles and provides the opportunity to overlay the Nordic walking technique on trekking.

TWO

The Benefits Of Nordic Walking

The potential of Nordic walking to positively benefit health, fitness and wellbeing has been widely recognised and dozens of studies have been carried out to provide evidence to support this. In this chapter, I will present some of the science and evidence for how Nordic walking can help support a happy and healthy life.

Fitness and wellbeing

Nordic walking offers a huge range of general health, fitness and wellbeing benefits, both physical and mental, for people of all ages and fitness levels.

Weight loss, strength and fitness

For many of us, it's a constant battle to maintain a healthy weight. We know that our risk of diabetes, cancer and cardiovascular disease increases as our weight does and that exercise can help, but we often struggle to find something that we enjoy and which we can easily build into our lives.

Regular brisk walking is one of the best exercises for maintaining a healthy weight and Nordic walking offers faster results.[7] A six-month study comparing the effects of diet combined with walking versus Nordic walking showed that while both activities had a significant impact, that of Nordic walking was greater.[8] People's body mass index (BMI), waist size, total body fat and leg fat all dropped further, their arm and leg strength increased and their aerobic fitness gains were greater. Why? Because Nordic walking uses your whole body. Your arms and upper body as well as your legs work to propel you forward, meaning you use more muscle and burn more calories than regular walking. With good technique you can expect to use around 20% more calories than regular walk, but it could be as high as 46%.[9] If you're looking for an outdoor exercise where you can walk and talk, burn calories, trim your waist and tone your arms and legs, start Nordic walking.

Mental health

Being active is key to mental health – inactive people are three times more likely to suffer from depression.[10] Just being outdoors in a park or green space can significantly lower your stress hormone levels and getting outdoors during daylight hours encourages your brain to produce serotonin and melatonin, chemicals that improve mood and sleep.[11] Regularly walking with others can help with depression and with Nordic walking you get the added benefit of learning a new skill, one of the NHS's five steps to mental wellbeing.[12]

Most of us know from experience that exercise boosts mood, lowers stress and makes us feel more energetic and positive, but pain and lack of confidence can stop us from getting started. Nordic walking is 'exercising easy'. The poles are fun to use, make you go faster, provide additional support, help with balance and generally make walking feel more energised. Your whole body moves and that feels good. In a nation-wide Nordic walking and mental wellbeing survey I conducted in 2021, 95% of respondents said that it had improved their mood, and over 80% said it had reduced their stress levels.

Ageing

By being physically active you reduce your chance of dying early by nearly a third.[13] It's that significant. You don't have to go to the gym or do anything dramatic. The simple act of walking in a way that raises your heart rate is sufficient.

Nordic walking is effective at increasing your heart rate because using your arms and upper body as well as your legs to move you forwards means your heart has to work harder. You don't even have to walk fast to benefit. Studies have shown that Nordic walking automatically increases your heart rate and oxygen uptake more than regular walking.[14] In summary, Nordic walking helps you to keep active and strong and research is consistently finding that it helps you to continue everyday activities and maintain your quality of life when you're older.

Joints and arthritis

I have had first-hand experience of the transformation Nordic walking can lead to for someone with sore joints and I have seen many of my clients benefitting too, especially those with hip and knee pain. Nordic walking mobilises joints throughout your body, keeping them lubricated and boosting the health of your cartilage. It supports your weight and encourages better posture. It also strengthens the muscles, ligaments and tendons surrounding your joints. These work together, protecting your joints and lessening pressure. If you've sore joints, Nordic walking can both relieve pain and help you walk farther.[15]

Aside from all these physiological benefits, Nordic walking is highly sociable. Participants in arthritis Nordic walking studies have said that the group nature of Nordic walking, having people there to support and keep you motivated even through those difficult moments, made all the difference.[16] In a continuing theme, one study looking at the benefits of Nordic walking for inflammatory rheumatic disease especially noted that everyone who had taken part in the research kept on Nordic walking together even after the project was over.[17]

Back pain

Until recently, back pain was mostly treated with painkillers and anti-inflammatory drugs like ibuprofen, but these have been shown to provide little benefit. One particularly striking review of thirty-five trials involving more than six thousand people found that only one in six patients received any pain-relieving benefit they would not have got from a placebo. They were also more than twice as likely to get stomach ulcers and other gut problems.[18]

The first recommendation of the NHS for treating back pain is to stay as active as possible. Taking up Nordic walking will positively impact your back health and studies have shown that you are likely to be able to walk with less pain and fewer muscle spasms when Nordic walking.[19,20] When done correctly, Nordic walking mobilises your back and strengthens the muscles around your spine. It also improves your balance and, thanks to the poles, the load on your spine, hips and knees is reduced. A twelve-week study following one hundred older adults with back, hip and/or knee pain recorded that 91% experienced a reduction in pain on walking (by an average of 80%) and an increase in the distance they were able to walk. When walking without poles, the pain on walking and the distance walked returned quickly to what they had been before. The study called on health providers to start recommending Nordic walking as an exercise for people with back, hip and knee pain.[21]

Osteoporosis and bone health

We need to pay attention to bone health because almost one in two women and one in five men over the age of fifty will break a bone, mainly due to poor bone health and conditions such as osteoporosis.[22]

Building exercise into our lives is one of the ways we can help keep our bones strong. Simply being physically active can reduce your chances of a hip fracture by 68%.[23] The whole-body nature of Nordic walking makes it an ideal weight-bearing, bone-strengthening exercise. Research supports this. In one study, post-menopausal pre-diabetic women Nordic walking two to three times a week were able to maintain their bone mass and density in their lower spine and thigh bone, while those in the control group who maintained their daily activities were not.[24] The denser your bones, the stronger they generally are and the less likely they are to break. The benefits extend to other risk fracture sites, like the arms. Neither walking nor jogging directly increases the load on your arms, Nordic walking does.[25] The movement of pushing the pole against the ground increases arm strength and improves bone density in this area. All in all, Nordic walking is a great exercise if you are worried about your bone health or managing osteoporosis.

Heart and circulation

By taking up an activity like Nordic walking you can reduce your risk of developing heart and circulatory diseases by as much as 35%.[26] Being active makes your heart physically stronger because your heart is a muscle. Exercise works and strengthens your heart just as it does other muscles in your body. It makes your heart wall healthier and increases the amount of blood your heart is able to pump with each beat. This improved efficiency allows your heart to beat slower, which in turn reduces your blood pressure. According to the British Heart Foundation, around 50% of all heart attacks and strokes are associated with high blood pressure.[27] It is one of the health risks that you can most easily change. Research shows that Nordic walking can improve your resting heart rate and your blood pressure.[28] A study with post-stroke patients recorded that functional mobility was significantly higher following treadmill programmes with poles than without.[29]

Nordic walking can also help with peripheral arterial disease (PAD), where you get cramping, aching or pain in your legs or hips while walking. A study funded by the British Heart Foundation compared Nordic walking with regular walking for PAD patients and found that the Nordic walking group could quickly walk farther than the regular walking group and that their gains were greater over twelve weeks.[30] A follow-up after one year showed that many participants kept on Nordic walking and that their maximum walking distance and speed continued to improve.

Health conditions

As well as general health and fitness benefits, Nordic walking is also associated with positive effects related to specific health conditions and diseases.

Cancer

Cancer not only causes direct harm and illness but, adding insult to injury, it comes with a whole package of treatment side effects. If you have cancer, you have probably already been told that exercise can reduce many of these side effects, including one of the most common and debilitating, cancer-related fatigue.[31] Neither rest nor sleep can shift this type of fatigue, but exercise, especially aerobic exercise, can. Something like Nordic walking can also help manage weight gain, rebuild your strength, reduce anxiety and improve your sleep.[32]

Studies have shown that Nordic walking is especially beneficial for those with breast cancer.[33] It can help you regain upper body strength and shoulder and arm mobility and can also help with lymphoedema, pain and swelling. Nordic walking improves physical fitness and supports emotional wellbeing, which can help to manage the depression that is often associated with breast cancer.

I have many years' experience establishing programmes and teaching Nordic walking to people with cancer. I have even spoken to King Charles about its benefits during a visit he made to the national cancer charity Penny Brohn UK. Nordic walking is holistic, supportive, safe and effective and can be a good friend and companion on your journey through cancer.

Dementia and Alzheimer's

Memory, how we think and speak, and how we feel and behave are a large part of our identity. Reading this book, for instance, and remembering its contents; recognising your loved ones and friends; engaging in lively conversation; recalling all the memories that amount to the story of your life. It's agonising witnessing the decline in these abilities of someone close to you.

Dementia and Alzheimer's are the leading cause of death in the UK – over one million of us are likely to have one of them by 2025.[34] You may feel helpless and at a loss for what to do, but while science hasn't yet found the answer, one thing scientists are confident about is that physical activity plays a key role in keeping our brains healthy. Exercise has a direct effect on the brain, boosting memory and thinking power, slowing cognitive decline and even promoting neurogenesis, the growth of new brain cells.[35]

The Alzheimer's Society says that of all the lifestyle changes that have been studied, taking regular physical exercise appears to be one of the best things you can do to reduce your risk of getting dementia.[36]

An exercise like Nordic walking that raises your heart rate and increases the blood flow to your brain reduces your risk of getting dementia by almost a third and helps slow the pace of decline if you already have it.[37]

Parkinson's

Just as it is for Alzheimer's, the Parkinson's Foundation says that, aside from taking medications on time, exercise is the single most important thing you can do to manage Parkinson's and lead the best possible life.[38] Although it is not a cure, exercise may help slow the progression of symptoms and can help with gait and balance, flexibility and posture, working memory and decision making, and quality of sleep.

You can probably think of all sorts of activities that fit the bill, but the benefits of walking, and especially Nordic walking, are impressive. This was made apparent in a study that compared the effects of a flexibility programme, walking and Nordic walking on Parkinson's symptoms.[39] It followed ninety patients over the course of six months. While pain, balance and quality of life were improved in all the groups, walking and Nordic walking improved stride length, walking pattern and speed, and overall fitness. Those that were part of the Nordic walking group showed the biggest gains, including in their posture and stability. The study made a point of highlighting that all those in the Nordic walking group continued the activity after the research ended.

While there is no one 'best' exercise, the benefits of Nordic walking are compelling, not least because it combines a skill-based exercise with an aerobic and muscle-strengthening activity. The fact that it's outdoors and is often done as a sociable group activity confers multiple other benefits. It's a perfect way to have a laugh, boost your mood and support your brain and body.

NIC'S STORY

I was diagnosed with Parkinson's aged forty-three but, looking back, I can recognise symptoms from around my mid-thirties. There are people diagnosed much younger than I was, it is not solely an older person's disease, and it affects people in different ways.

I continued working for about ten more years before I took retirement as the symptoms became progressively more difficult to deal with. I also had to stop sport, which was hard as I played many to a high standard. I probably went through a period of depression. I knew I was missing something, as I was not physically active, but I didn't know exactly what that could be.

Through my neurology team I became aware of Nordic walking and its reported benefits for people with Parkinson's. Close to where I lived there was a newly started Parkinson's Nordic walking group, including for partners and friends. I joined up and from day one I was out in front developing a rhythm for my dynamic movements, which I know can aid neurological recovery. Ensuring a good heel strike and rolling through my foot to my toes soon sorted a lazy right foot and being challenged to keep my head up addressed my posture (apparently, I have a natural, five-degree forward tilt). I built up my strength and stamina over increasing distance training sessions and within a year of starting, I Nordic walked the Bristol 10km in an hour and twenty-two minutes, passing a fair few runners.

As well as the physical side, the importance of the post-walk coffee and cake and camaraderie should not be forgotten. Walking in the park in all weathers, absorbing the vitamin D with like-minded people of dissimilar ability, who all shared a common issue, led to lasting friendships. It made me feel part of something good.

Diabetes

If you have diabetes or are at risk of it, you will probably know that exercising can make a positive difference. It helps you lose weight and directly increases your body's insulin sensitivity.[40] I would encourage you to consider Nordic walking if you have diabetes. It supports your body while at the same time raising your heart rate, working your muscles and burning calories. In one study of type two diabetic women, Nordic walking for twelve weeks in a structured programme enabled them to significantly reduce their average blood sugar levels (HbA1c), BMI, and weight.[41] The active heel/toe roll and arm swing of Nordic walking also boosts your circulation and improves the blood supply to your legs and feet, helping to prevent cramps and support foot health. The small addition of two poles when you walk could make a big difference to your diabetes.

SUMMARY OF PART ONE

By now, you should understand what Nordic walking is, the context in which it emerged and how it was developed. You know what the key differences are between Nordic walking and regular walking, running and trekking, which relate chiefly to the whole-body nature of the workout you get, and why Nordic walking poles are not the same as trekking poles. You know about the breadth of research supporting the benefits of Nordic walking for fitness, wellbeing and overall health, as well as for many specific conditions ranging from cancer to diabetes, to Parkinson's disease. We've learned that it is the perfect activity to meet your exercise needs throughout your life, with many specific benefits as you age, including supporting and strengthening painful or weak joints and bones.

PART TWO

THE FOUR STEPS TO NORDIC WALKING SUCCESS

This part of the book will take you through four simple steps to Nordic walking success – posture, breathing, walking action, and active use of poles – and why they're important for your health. Along the way, I'll share technique tips, mistakes to avoid and some useful exercises. At the end of each section is a link to a short video explaining how to put what you've learned into practice. By the end of this part, you will know the basics of Nordic walking and be ready to get started. If you are already a Nordic walker, this part will be a useful refresher and offer extra pointers.

THREE

Step One: Posture

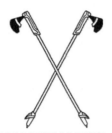

How you hold your body can have a profound impact, not only on your health, but also on shaping your self-image and self-confidence. Once your skeleton is properly aligned, your body is able to function more efficiently, your breathing becomes easier and deeper, your muscles less tense, your circulation improves and your joints become less stressed and vulnerable. Plus, you'll feel taller (because you are) and your chest and waist won't be so scrunched.

Nordic walking not only helps you walk with correct posture, but it also strengthens your postural muscles, meaning that you continue to benefit long after your Nordic walk is over. This is particularly important in today's world where almost everything seems bent on pulling you out of position. Sitting, driving, texting, or typing on a poorly set up computer all place stress on your neck, shoulders and lower back, encourage your head to jut forwards and your chest to slump.

Nordic walking cannot undo structural alterations due to factors like age-related wear and tear, injury, surgery, or birth misalignment, so don't try to force yourself into what you think is the 'perfect' position. Give yourself time, pay attention to the technique and allow your body to naturally recalibrate itself.

If you have an existing condition (like a shoulder impingement), Nordic walking is best used in conjunction with physiotherapy, at least to begin with. The Nordic walking loosens and strengthens and the physiotherapy deals with the underlying condition. Once this has been resolved, Nordic walking then becomes your ongoing maintenance activity. This is great news for you, as it's fun as well as effective.

Spine

Your spine is literally your body's backbone, its central supporting structure. It holds you up, enables you to move and protects a key part of your central nervous system, your spinal cord. Your spine is made up of bones (vertebrae), shock-absorbing discs separating the vertebrae, ligaments, and muscles. They can all be positively impacted by physical activity, and an exercise like Nordic walking is great for your spine.

Nordic walking with good spine alignment doesn't mean trying to alter the shape of your spine, you are simply trying to expand the gaps. Collapsed down, your vertebrae and discs weigh on one another. They have no energy. If you can expand the spaces between them, lifting them up and off one another, you allow them to move freely and flex. Once your vertebrae are no longer compacted, your spine is able to return to its natural soft S shape (sideways on, there are gentle spinal curves at your neck and lower back) and your shock-absorbing discs have space to plump up and do their job more efficiently. Once you introduce a gentle rotation your spine will be re-energised.

Top tips

⬭ **Imagine your spine is like an accordion**, the musical instrument that expands as you pull it open. Expand the spaces between your vertebrae, lifting them up and off one another, taking the pressure off your discs.

⬭ **Lengthen your spine** up the back of your neck, so that the back of your head lifts upward toward the sky.

Common mistakes

⬭ **Lengthening vertically** but leaning to one side.

Head

Your head is extremely heavy. It weighs in at around 5kg (10–12lbs), which is like balancing five standard bags of sugar on your shoulders. Every inch your head juts forward can put an additional 10lbs (4.5kg) of weight on your spine.[42,43] This means that if your head is not perfectly stacked (particularly common these days, when so many people suffer from 'text neck') your whole body can be pulled out of shape, putting pressure on your neck, causing stress and tension and reducing your lung capacity.[44]

The perfect head position is where, front on, your head is not tilting to one side and, sideways on, your ears sit above your shoulders. This won't happen straight away if your head has been out of alignment for many years, but following these tips, especially while walking will help encourage it back towards its proper place.

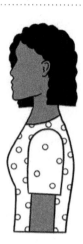

Top tips

- **Imagine there's a helium balloon tied to the top of the back of your head**, lifting your head up and off your shoulders. At the same time, drop your shoulders down.

- **Slide your chin back** (think double chin) so that your ears move back toward sitting above your shoulders, but only do this as far as feels comfortable.

- **Keep your chin parallel with the ground.**

- **Keep your neck relaxed**, wobble your head occasionally to check tension hasn't built up in your neck.

- **Relax your jaw.**

Common mistakes

- **Lifting the front of your head.** This tips your head backward and results in compression rather than lengthening of the vertebrae in your neck.

- **Looking at your feet.** Scan the ground with your eyes but keep your head up. If you can see your feet when you are walking, you have dropped your head. With a correct head position, you should only see them peek into your peripheral vision.

- **Lifting your shoulders up with your head.**

- **Tense neck, clenched jaw.**

Shoulders and chest

The tasks and worries of modern daily living encourage us to round our shoulders forward and up toward our ears, creating tightness and tension, weakened back muscles, cramped lung space and a reduced ability to swing our arms correctly. Rounded shoulders and a tight chest are a bad double act. If you get one, you'll almost certainly get the other – and you want neither. Your upper back and head are directly affected by the position of your chest. If your chest is slumped, your spine will be excessively rounded, your back muscles will weaken, your head will push forward and your neck will tighten. You want to keep your chest lifted, not only to improve your posture, but because your rib cage houses your heart and lungs, so if space there is confined your breathing and oxygen availability will be compromised.

In short, poor shoulder and chest alignment play havoc with the smooth running of your body and lead to a stooped posture as you age. Below are my top tips for good shoulder and chest posture:

Top tips

- **Roll your shoulders back** and down away from your ears.

- **Slide the base of your shoulder blades (your 'angel wings') towards each other.**

- **Stand tall**, out of your hips, lengthening the gap between your hip bone and rib cage – imagine you have a spring between your hip bone and rib cage that stops your chest collapsing down.

- **Puff your chest out** so that it sits proud. It should be the first part of your body to bump into an object in front of you.

Common mistakes

- **Rounding your shoulders forward.**

- **Allowing your chest to slump down.**

- **Lifting your shoulders up** as you lift your chest up.

Hips and pelvis

At the bottom of your spine sits your pelvis, with your hips at the front and your sacrum at the back. The position of your pelvis affects the curve at the base of your spine, which is a common area for back ache. The pelvis is directly affected by how tight the muscles around it are, especially your hip flexors at the front (used for sitting), your hamstrings up the back of your thigh and your glutes in your buttocks.

Walking with your hips correctly levelled can help reduce lower back pain and re-instate the correct amount of curve, enabling your spinal curves to work in harmony for optimum weight bearing, shock absorption and flexibility. I know that it's not always possible to have completely level hips (if you've scoliosis or one leg shorter than the other, for example), but these tips will hopefully help you achieve the best pelvic position for your body:

Top tips

- **Your pelvis should sit in a level position**, neither tipped forward (giving you an excessive lower back arch) nor backward (giving you a flat lower back). Imagine balancing a tray on the top of your pelvis with full glasses of water that you don't want to spill.

- **Gently engage your tummy muscles just below your belly button**, by pulling them in toward your spine.

- **Push through your hips and squeeze your glutes** as you push off with your toes. You should feel a stretch at the top of your thigh or in the hip flexor itself if you're doing it right.

Common mistakes

- *Sticking your bottom too far back.* This pulls your lower back into an excessive curve and puts added pressure on your spine.

- *Flattening your lower back* so that there's no curve and no room for your spine to compress to absorb the weight of your upper body.

- *Dropping one hip down/hitching it up as you walk* (it is sometimes not possible to avoid this, depending on your body's structure).

- *Not using your hamstrings and glutes for walking.*

Your glutes

Your gluteal muscles ('glutes') are a set of three muscles located in each buttock. The biggest of these is the gluteus maximus. After your heart, it has the honour of being the largest and most powerful muscle in your body.

Each set of glutes work together to move the hip and thigh of the leg they're attached to, which means that they're involved with practically every action of your lower body – walking, sitting and climbing stairs to name a few. They stabilise your pelvis and spine, prevent injury and enable you to walk faster. You would think that such an important group of muscles would tend to work properly, but your glutes are like a grumpy teenager – they switch off easily, once asleep are difficult to wake and even when awake might not function correctly. Sitting down for long periods, a previous injury, postural imbalance or structural issues like having one leg longer than the other can all impact how well your glutes work. If they are not working properly, your clever body reroutes and gets other muscles – such as your back, thighs and hamstrings – to do the work instead. But these muscles are not designed for the job, which causes all sorts of problems, from back ache to knee and foot problems and even shoulder and shin pains.

Another reason your glutes might not be working properly is if you have tight hip flexors. Hip flexors are a group of deep muscles that connect your legs to your pelvis. When you bend your knee or bend from your hips, you use your hip flexors. Tight hip flexors and weak glutes often go together. Again, the chief culprit is sitting down too much (many adults spend over 7 hours per day).[45] Sitting shortens your hip flexors at the front of your hips and stretches your glutes in your buttocks. The longer you spend sitting, the shorter and weaker, respectively, these muscles become, de-stabilising your hips/pelvis and compromising the long-term mobility, stability and safety of your lower body and back.

The wonderful thing is that just by walking with good technique (which Nordic walking teaches), you can strengthen your glutes, stretch your hip flexors and contribute to a stable lower body and back.

HOW CAN YOU TELL IF YOUR GLUTES AREN'T WORKING PROPERLY?

It's not always possible to self-diagnose whether your glutes are functioning fully. To do this, you would need to go to a physio or other health professional who could run a series of functional tests. But there is a fun little test you can do yourself, which goes like this:

1. Stand with your feet hip width apart, tummy pulled in, hands on your bottom.

2. Squeeze one buttock and then the other (you should feel your hand move when it tightens).

What happened? Could you squeeze each buttock in isolation or did the other want to join in as well? Were both sides as strong as each other, or could you squeeze one side better? Even if you could isolate each buttock, this doesn't mean that they will perform properly when you start to move.

Posture Video link:
https://letswalknordic.com/nordic-walking/how-to-videos/#posture

FOUR

Step Two: Breathing

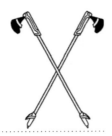

Breath is life. It brings us oxygen and provides the energy our bodies need to function. But because breathing is automatic it's not something most of us consciously think about and many of us don't breathe correctly. We either breathe too quickly and shallowly, or we breathe with our upper chest and not our diaphragm. It's also common to unconsciously hold your breath for extended periods. Breathing changes when we are in different emotional states. When we're stressed or nervous, we tend to take fast and shallow breaths; when we're relaxed, we breathe more steadily and deeply.

Disrupted breathing patterns cause all sorts of problems, aside from starving your body of oxygen. In particular, your neck and shoulder muscles have to work super hard to help your lungs pull air in, causing them to be in a perpetual state of tension. This tension will pull on your spine, collarbone and base of your skull, which distorts your posture and often leads to headaches and pain.

Nordic walking is a perfect opportunity to improve your breathing. Not only do you generally not out-walk your breath, but its rhythmic nature encourages and supports a healthy breathing pattern. It's a mutually beneficial relationship – breathing well improves your Nordic walking, and Nordic walking will improve your breathing.

'Breathing well' means pulling fresh air into your lungs and pushing stale air out. Your diaphragm is the main muscle involved in this. It sits like an umbrella under your ribs. When it moves down, it creates suction to draw in air and expand your lungs; when it moves up, it pushes the old air out. Your diaphragm should be doing about 80% of the work when you breathe.

Breathing diaphragmatically also supports your lymphatic system, which is part of your immune system and helps protect you from disease. Just as the heart is the pump for the circulatory system, the diaphragm contributes to the movement of lymph (the fluid that carries your infection-fighting, antibody-producing white blood cells) around your body. Another way in which lymph moves around your body is through your own movement, so an activity like Nordic walking which moves both your upper and lower body plus encourages diaphragmatic breathing will greatly support your immune system.

Top Tips

- **Diaphragm breathe** (otherwise known as 'belly breathing') by gently nudging your belly out as you breathe in, drawing air in like you're inflating a balloon. Aim to fill your belly with air first, your lower ribs second and your upper chest last (you might not get that far).

- **Breathe in through your nose** where possible. This warms or cools and filters the air. Breathe out through either your nose or mouth.

- **Breathe out for a little longer than you breathe in.**

- **Use the rhythm of your walking** to create a consistent breathing pattern. Count your breath in and out.

- **Your head, shoulders and chest posture** are crucial for good breathing.

Common mistakes

- **Breathing in through your mouth** (unless you have to).

- **Slouching.**

- **Lifting your shoulders as you breathe in.** Keep them rolled back, down and relaxed.

LUNG FACTS

Your lungs mature by the time you are around twenty-five and the average lung capacity of a healthy adult is about six litres.[46] Your lung function decreases as you age but good posture, good breathing technique and exercise all help to keep your lungs healthy.

HEATHER'S STORY

I was diagnosed with asthma out of the blue after feeling low and ill for some months. It was the perfect excuse to avoid exercise for fear of breathlessness. I managed my asthma by self-limiting my exercise. My weight increased progressively, especially following (on separate occasions) the incapacity of a broken foot, fractured toes and torn cartilage in my knee.

Following recovery from foot surgery, I heard about Nordic walking from a colleague and signed up for an induction course. I quickly noticed the health benefits: improved fitness; less breathlessness; an improvement in my walking and posture; and an overall sense of achievement. I combined my walking with a healthy eating programme. My weight started to drop and the more walking sessions I did, the more I wanted to do. I felt fit, healthy and naturally energised.

My asthma has receded to the extent that I no longer use steroid or reliever inhalers and, although not yet confirmed by my GP, I feel it has resolved. I am not afraid of the challenge of exercise; I now embrace it and am looking forward to participating in a Nordic walking marathon, something I would not have contemplated eighteen months ago.

Nordic walking ticks all the boxes for me: the de-stressing and the sense of wellbeing, my improved breathing and fitness and, not be underestimated, its sociable nature and the friendships I have developed.

My friends and family laugh at how I have even overcome a pathological fear of mud. I'm now quite happy sloshing over muddy fields and through swampy bridle paths in pursuit of the pure enjoyment of Nordic walking.

Breathing Video link:
https://letswalknordic.com/nordic-walking/how-to-videos/#breathing

FIVE

Step Three: Walking Action

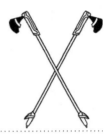

Walking is fundamental to our lives. We've been doing it for so long that we generally don't think about what's involved in putting one foot in front of the other, but it's a surprisingly complicated movement and can easily be done poorly.

To walk correctly, many things need to work in unison: good posture, correct muscle activation, using your arms and feet properly and good balance. Once sloppy habits have been formed, it's hard to unscramble them unless something like Nordic walking acts as a trigger for change.

Feet

Besides taking your whole weight when you are standing or walking, feet have a lot to put up with. Most of us have at least one foot that turns out or in as we walk, and foot pain, stiff ankles, badly fitting shoes, corns, calluses and bunions can all alter the way we walk. Conditions like diabetes or treatments for cancer and other medications can also affect the feet.

One of the most conspicuous aspects of walking is the way we use (or rather don't use) our feet and ankles. Look around you and you'll see that many people have a passive foot strike, where their foot hits the ground more or less flat instead of articulating from the heel to the toes. Over time, a passive foot strike results in your ankle and foot becoming less and less pliable. The shin muscles then weaken, walking turns into shuffling and trips and falls will likely follow.

Nordic walking is one of few activities that requires us to think about our foot action. Walking correctly means actively articulating your foot, rolling from the heel through to your toes in a smooth action. It's a great way to keep the joints and muscles in and around your feet healthy and it's especially important as you age and your skin thins and joints begin to stiffen.

Top tips

- **Lift your toes toward your knee as you step forward.** Your heel will then naturally drop softly to the ground. Lifting your toes strengthens your shin muscle and reduces your risk of tripping. It also helps pump the blood back up your leg to your heart, keeping your circulation strong. This is especially beneficial if you have varicose veins.

- **The underneath of your foot has three rockers** to help move you forward: your heel, your forefoot and your toes. Use those rockers to propel you forward by rolling actively through your foot from your heel to your toes in a fluid action.

- **As you rock over your toes, raise your heel and push your thigh back.** If you're doing it properly, you will feel a stretch at the top of your thigh and (if your shoes are flexible enough) across the top of your foot. Your ankle will be 'open'.

- **Spread your toes wide**, like a duck's webbed feet.

- **Keep your weight evenly balanced over both feet.**

- **Tread lightly over the ground** using your tummy muscles to control your foot fall. (Refer back to Step One – Posture for how to engage these muscles.)

- **If your feet point out, think 'middle toe' as you push off.** You might also try rotating your entire leg in toward your centre line so that your knee and foot are pointing more forward. Only do this as much as feels comfortable; speak to a biomechanics expert if you want to correct a turned-out foot posture.

Common mistakes

- **Wearing badly fitting shoes.**

- **Ignoring pain in your feet.**

- **Being over-active with your feet** if you have foot arthritis.

- **Shifting your weight to one side as you walk.**

- **Bouncing upward** as you push off with your toes. You want your energy moving forward not upward.

- **Scrunching your toes.**

- **Over-striding.** Always take normal steps.

EXPERT VIEW: NAOMI GREEN, PODIATRIST – FACTS ABOUT FEET

1. How we walk and look after our feet hugely influences their health. Using them properly will improve your circulation, ankle stability and balance.

2. We have a whopping twenty-six bones, thirty-three joints and nineteen muscles in each foot (twenty-nine combined with the muscles in the leg that cross over the ankle into the foot and help position the foot), all of which need to be mobilised, strengthened and stretched to keep healthy.

3. Poorly fitting shoes that are too tight on the toes can damage your feet and affect the performance of your whole body.

4. It is worth doing regular exercises (in addition to Nordic walking) to help the strength, flexibility and condition of your feet and their combined sixty-six joints. These are most effective when done shoeless. Good exercises include lifting a pencil with your toes; walking on tiptoes and on your heels; rolling your feet over a tennis or spikey massage ball.

5. The right socks are almost as important as the right shoes. Our feet have 250,000 sweat glands, which can produce up to half a pint of perspiration daily.

Arms

An important but often forgotten component in the process of walking is your arm swing. It's an integral and essential part of both walking and Nordic walking and is simple and intuitive, yet lots of us don't swing our arms much when we walk. I'm not sure why. Maybe it's because we're holding phones or shopping bags or we've got into the habit of walking with our hands in our pockets.

Swinging your arms helps keep your circulation flowing effectively and your shoulder joints (among the most complicated joints in the body) mobile. It can also be used as an accelerator. Swinging your arm supports your lymphatic and immune system and is important for head stability and general balance.[47,48] Even if you have a sore shoulder or the common rotator cuff injury, the forward-backward movement of Nordic walking seems to be manageable for most people, enabling them to generate power without triggering discomfort.

Top tips

- **Your shoulders need to be wide** for your arms to swing freely. Lift your chest and roll your shoulders back and down, keeping them relaxed.

- **Your arm swing should come from your shoulder first**, with a soft bend from your elbow second. It's a pendulum movement and should feel natural and comfortable.

- **Your arms and legs should move in harmony**, with the opposite arm and leg going forward at the same time.

- **If you want to walk faster, speed up your arm swing.**

- **The palms of your hands should face inward at all times.**

Common mistakes

- *Swinging your arms across the vertical midline of your body.*

- *Lifting your shoulders up as you swing your arms.*

- *Slouching or rounding your shoulders* forward, as this will inhibit a free arm swing.

- *Hinging at your elbow.*

- *Holding your arms out to the side*, away from your body. They should hang and swing nice and close to your body but not actually brushing your side.

MICHAEL'S STORY

I picked up a bilateral rotator cuff injury about eighteen months ago, which was diagnosed as impingement syndrome. I had extensive treatment with a chiropractor and physio, which seemed to make things worse. My right shoulder recovered on its own, but my left shoulder didn't. Then I started Nordic walking and initially my shoulder would be tight and painful, especially during warm up and cool down.

As the months went by, I kept hearing about keeping the shoulders low, the torso ready to rotate and to push through the hand strap, and I found myself concentrating on these three things. Initially, I didn't notice much of a difference, but then my shoulder gradually started to feel looser, although it was still tight and painful at times. I continued to concentrate on keeping my shoulders down and relaxed, and on the torso twist.

I had some further physio, this time from a more experienced practitioner who had dealt with a lot of shoulder injuries, and he was fascinated by the Nordic walking. He could see how it would be beneficial and gave me exercises that targeted not my bad shoulder as such, but my shoulder girdle and core muscles. I've since been discharged from the physio as things have improved massively.

I've noticed that:

- As my shoulder became looser, I was pushing back through the hand straps more efficiently and my shoulder movement became more fluid.

- As my torso rotation improved, my shoulder released and I stood taller and less rounded.

- During cool down stretches, I can now get the poles behind my head and onto the back of my shoulders – I couldn't do this when I started and although I could raise my arm above my head, it was painful. Now it's pain free.

- I can also do the exercise with the poles vertically down the back. Previously, my left shoulder was too tight to pull down or up without pain and I had trouble reaching the poles.

HOW CAN YOU TELL IF YOU HAVE SHOULDER IMPINGEMENT?

Shoulder injury or impingement is a big issue for many, and it can creep up on you, developing gradually over time. Ask yourself these questions:

1. Is my shoulder stiff?

2. Am I able to move my arm in every direction (up/down, in/out, full circles backward and forward)?

3. Can I do straps and zips up behind my back?

4. Does my shoulder feel a bit unstable, like it could pop or slide out of the socket?

5. Does my shoulder seem to lack strength when I try and lift things, especially above my head?

If the answer to any of the above is 'yes', then maybe your shoulders need some care and attention from a trained professional. Happily, one of the by-products of good Nordic walking technique is improved shoulder health and increased mobility.

Rotate

Did you know that your spine is designed to gently rotate as you walk? Your lower body (from where your bottom rib attaches to your spine) moves one way as you step forward and your upper body is designed to twist the other way. This subtle movement is one of the least known but most valuable of all the movements your spine makes. It boosts circulation the whole way down your spine and increases oxygen and nutrients to your inter-vertebral discs. It also strengthens the small connecting muscles between your vertebrae. In traditional Chinese medicine, this twist point where the thoracic spine meets the lumbar spine is one of the main points where chi (energy) enters the body. It also happens to be the point where your diaphragm attaches to your spine.

If you don't already naturally rotate your upper body (that's most of us), this is one of the hardest movements to learn. It's well worth practising and one of the easiest ways to do this is at home standing in front of a mirror. Learn how with my top tips below:

Top tips

- **Roll your shoulders back and down.**

- **Gently pull the base of your shoulder blades together.**

- **Keep your neck relaxed.**

- **As you swing your arm backward**, try to slide your shoulder blade diagonally down and across, as though you are trying to post it in your opposite back trouser pocket. Maybe even imagine a rope is tied to the bottom of each shoulder blade, pulling like you would a bell down toward your opposite buttock.

- **Use the momentum of your arm** swinging backward to twist your rib cage with it. To practise this in front of a mirror, place one foot forward, keeping your hips and belly button still and rotate your upper body left to right. Your chest and shoulders should move one way then the other. Don't forget to switch legs and don't force it – it's a gentle movement.

Common mistakes

- **Tensing your neck and shoulders.** Keep them relaxed. Wobble your head on your shoulders every so often and make sure your head is sitting properly over your body (refer back to Step One – Posture for the correct head positioning).

- **Dipping your shoulders down to the side.** Your shoulders should be level.

- **Hitching each hip up as you walk.** Again, your hips should be level.

- **Rounding your shoulders forward.** Rolling your shoulders back and down every so often is a good habit to get into.

- **Rotating too much.** You only need a gentle movement to get the health benefits.

Walking Action Video link:
https://letswalknordic.com/nordic-walking/how-to-videos/#walking-action

SIX

Step Four: Active Use Of Poles

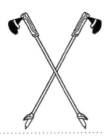

This is the most exciting part of Nordic walking as using poles in the correct way engages your torso, arms and shoulders, and you can feel your whole body walking, not just your legs. Unless you've Nordic walked before, it will be a completely new experience so it's best if you can learn from an instructor. However, if that's not possible, here are my four golden rules and top tips for using Nordic walking poles correctly.

1. Use the right height poles

It might seem obvious, but using poles that are the wrong length for you will affect the quality of your technique and the benefit you get from Nordic walking. Too short and you won't feel that upper body resistance or be able to swing your arms fully for maximum power and propulsion. Too long and your technique will be compromised, placing stress on your muscles, especially in your neck and shoulders. The ideal pole height is when, holding the pole vertically beside you, your forearm is horizontal or slightly lower than horizontal.

As your technique, posture and range of motion improve, you may well want a longer pole to get greater propulsion. It's why I recommend adjustable poles to most clients when they first start out. Even experienced Nordic walkers might want to adjust their poles depending on the terrain they're walking on. You can read more about poles in chapter seven on kit.

2. Always angle your poles backward

Angling the poles backward immediately puts your body in better alignment and helps you walk faster. If you push down on poles held vertically you just push yourself up toward the sky, but if you angle your poles backward and push you'll go forward. The same amount of effort is required. You are just being more efficient with how you use the poles.

Angling the poles backward also minimises the possibility of tripping over your poles. Fear of tripping with poles attached to your hands is probably the main reason people are put off Nordic walking. If you always angle the poles backward and use your arms correctly (see rule three below) you will be planting them by your back foot, so you shouldn't ever get tangled up with your feet.

3. Swing your arm from your shoulder

Not swinging your arm properly is one of the most common mistakes Nordic walkers make. Nordic walking requires the same arm swing as regular walking but with more zing. I've already said it, but it's worth repeating, swing from your shoulder, don't clamp your upper arm into your side and hinge from your elbow. If you do, you will be missing out on many of the health benefits and will probably get a sore elbow too.

Swinging from the shoulder doesn't mean you need to keep your arm rigidly straight. On the contrary, as you swing your arm forward it will naturally bend slightly. This is correct, it's called a 'soft' elbow. Some people have more of a soft elbow than others, which is fine so long as it doesn't develop into an elbow hinge.

A good arm swing is one that has a steady pendulum rhythm. As your arm strength increases, you should be able to extend your backswing behind your hip, generating more power and significantly increasing your upper body workout.

4. Push through the strap

Your arm push is key to your success with Nordic walking. Actively pushing through the strap down to the tip of the pole engages your upper body muscles and allows you to swing your arm more fully, giving you greater power and enabling you to use your whole body. It's why trekking poles, with their thin looped straps, aren't suitable for Nordic walking. The more firmly you push through the strap, and the longer you maintain that downward pressure as you swing your arm backward, the more you'll tone your arms and shoulders.

Make sure the strap fits your hand snugly to enable a smooth transfer of power. Relax your hand grip as you push the pole backward and gently squeeze your hand round the grip (as though you were shaking someone's hand) as you swing your arm forward. Eventually you will be able to power the pole way behind your body, letting go of the handle completely and snapping your hand closed round the grip as you swing forward.

Putting it all together

Combined, the four golden rules above will enable you to get to grips – literally – with Nordic walking poles and start you on your journey.

If you're new to Nordic walking, you might find that one side of your body is weaker and less co-ordinated than the other and that you struggle to get the same control and clean pole plant. This is perfectly normal. Most of us have a dominant side and it takes a while for our brains and hands to synchronise and achieve a smooth and efficient action. One of the benefits of Nordic walking is that it strengthens both sides of your body, leaving you better balanced. Excellent exercises for improving your use of the poles include:

- Single-arm poling, where you Nordic walk with one pole only (carrying the other). This allows you to concentrate on one side at a time, which is much easier.

- Double-arm poling, where both arms and hands are doing the same thing at the same time.

- If you're having trouble co-ordinating your arms and legs, let go of the poles completely and allow them to drag along the ground beside you as you walk and swing your arms, basically pretending they're not there. It's like hitting the reset button and you'll start walking correctly again in no time.

Active Use Of Poles Video link:
https://letswalknordic.com/nordic-walking/how-to-videos/#active-use-of-poles

SUMMARY OF PART TWO

To begin with, you will have to consciously remember the Nordic walking foundations, but gradually they will slip into your subconscious so that when you pick up your poles you will automatically stand taller with better posture and walk and breathe correctly. Even better, you'll eventually assimilate it into your regular walking and your balance, posture, joints, circulation and lower body tone will improve dramatically even without the poles. The key take-aways from this part of the book and things to keep in mind are:

- Your posture – head up, eyes down, chest proud, tummy in, shoulders down and relaxed.

- Your breathing – in through your nose if possible, inflating your belly and lower ribs first, in rhythm with your walking.

- Your lower body – active feet, engaged leg and buttock muscles (glutes) and open, lifted hips.

- The angle of your pole – it should be about 45 degrees from vertical.

- Where you're planting your pole – by your back foot.

- How you are pushing into your pole – your arm should be straight with a 'soft' elbow, shoulders down, pushing through the strap down to the tip of the pole and engaging your triceps (tops of the back of your arms).

PART THREE

MAKING NORDIC WALKING WORK FOR YOU

To get the most from Nordic walking you need more than just correct technique. This chapter explains what kit you need for Nordic walking, the different types of poles available and what's best for you. You will also learn how much exercise is enough and what level of intensity you should be striving for, based on your age and health status. I'll give you a simple method for measuring your exercise intensity, as well as explaining how and when to increase intensity and how to set clear and achievable goals. I always begin my Nordic walks with some warm-ups and finish with stretches and I will share with you my top ten of each so that you can ready your body and make sure it's well balanced at the end. I will also provide practical tips on how to Nordic walk over different terrain, including slopes and hills, muddy ground and tarmac.

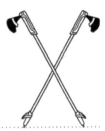

SEVEN

Kit

The only specialist kit you need for Nordic walking is a pair of Nordic walking poles. Besides the poles, it's helpful to have shoes or boots with a flexible sole and clothing that's comfortable and breathable. But first up, let's talk about the all-important Nordic walking poles. What do they look like and how do they work?

Nordic walking poles

It's important that you don't accidentally buy trekking poles for Nordic walking because you won't get the same benefits and will place stress on your wrists and forearms if you use them with the Nordic walking technique. Nordic walking poles are simple in design, but like any piece of equipment the quality and price varies. There are three components to a Nordic walking pole: the handle and glove-type strap, the shaft, and the tip and paw (rubber pad) at the bottom.

The glove-type strap of Nordic walking poles is one of the key features that set them apart from trekking poles. Its unique design prevents over-gripping, which stresses the muscles of your forearm, neck and shoulders, and allows you to push through the strap to activate your arms and upper body. Some manufacturers offer small, medium and large straps for different hand sizes and you can also buy straps integrated into a full or half glove. These are useful if you have arthritic hands as it helps to spread the load, making it more comfortable to push through the strap. Most straps have a release button or trigger mechanism that detaches them from the pole handle. The handle itself is slender so that it can slide through your hand easily as you push the pole back. It can be made from rubber or other materials, but most often it will have a cork grip, which is non-slip, is nice to touch and absorbs sweat.

The shaft of Nordic walking poles is generally carbon, aluminium, or a mix of the two. Aluminium poles are cheaper and a sensible choice if you're only Nordic walking occasionally. Carbon is lighter than aluminium and absorbs more of the vibration when the pole strikes the ground. It's really a question of budget. Carbon is pricier, but even the most expensive Nordic walking poles are cheap compared with golf clubs, tennis racquets and most other sports equipment.

The paw is the stopper at the base of the pole. On Nordic walking poles, it is angled so that you get good grip without compromising your technique. Underneath is the tip, which is usually made from a strong metal such as tungsten carbide. Some tips are blunt, others sharply pointed. Generally, you have the paw on when walking on hard surfaces and the paw removed when on soft surfaces, as this enables the tip to dig into the ground and give you extra purchase.

The advantages and disadvantages of different Nordic pole types

Type of pole	Advantages	Disadvantages
Fixed length (one piece) pole No adjustment areas	Reliable Feels nice to use (good 'swing' weight) No vibration with top-quality carbon poles Often comes with a speed spike tip, which digs into the ground well and supports good technique	You need to know your exact length – there's no room for adjustment Poles are sold in 5cm increments (100–130cm) and you might be an 'in-between' size You can't easily travel with them. As your technique and/or posture improves, you may want a longer pole, so not ideal for beginners
Adjustable pole One adjustment either in the middle of the shaft (called an 'adjustable' pole) or near the top (called an 'extendable' pole)	More portable than fixed poles but won't fit in a suitcase Good if you: Don't know what length pole you need Want to share your poles with others Want flexibility to change your pole length	Adjustable poles will generally have more vibration than fixed length poles, which is especially noticeable on hard ground The adjustment point is a potential weak point and the tightening mechanism can sometimes get stuck or break
Travel pole A three-piece pole with two adjustment/break points	Portable, especially the foldable poles Foldable poles are very light	The same disadvantages as adjustable poles Foldable poles are expensive

Pole length

Nordic walking poles can be bought in or adjusted to different lengths. The correct length for you will depend on your height, technique, the terrain you're walking on and your body's natural mobility and stability. When holding the pole vertically beside you with your elbow tucked into your side, your forearm should be bent at a 90-degree angle or slightly greater. The textbook formula for working out the right pole length is your height in centimetres multiplied by 0.68. But there are many variables that can affect this, especially when you're starting out and perfecting the technique, so unless you are an experienced Nordic walker and know your exact pole length, I would recommend buying adjustable poles. Most people, when they start Nordic walking, find it easier to use a shorter pole, but as technique and strength improve a longer pole will give more resistance and involve your arms and upper body more. Adjustable poles give you the option to alter your pole length as you progress.

Choosing between fixed length, adjustable or travel poles for Nordic walking depends mostly on what you want to use them for and also on your budget. There is no one pole that's perfect for every occasion. Foldable and travel poles are fabulous in many respects but their tip systems mean they aren't well suited for winter walking in the UK – and they are expensive. Fixed/adjustable poles aren't very portable. A special word of caution if flying: your poles are likely to be confiscated if you take them in your cabin luggage, so always put them in the hold.

Clothing

While you don't need specialist or specific 'fitness' clothing to enjoy Nordic walking, some consideration of what you're wearing on your upper and lower body, and of course your feet, will enable you to get the most out of your walking and avoid any discomfort.

Body

Layering clothing on your upper body gives you the versatility you need for Nordic walking. On a cold day, you may start off feeling chilly at the beginning of a walk, but you will certainly warm up once you get going. Layering several layers of lighter clothing will provide sufficient warmth while enabling you to easily remove (and carry) light layers as you warm up. In winter, you will probably want a base layer, followed by a fleece or similar as the mid-layer, under a jacket as your top layer. All your layers should be made from breathable fabric to allow the heat and perspiration to wick away from your body and evaporate. It's best if they're not too bulky so that they don't restrict your movement and arm swing. I wouldn't recommend cotton as it absorbs moisture and can start to rub or make you feel cold once you slow down or stop.

On your lower body, you don't need any LYCRA® or leggings to Nordic walk, just something comfortable that allows freedom of movement. Most of my clients wear trousers, but shorts, skirts or even dresses are fine too so long as they don't restrict your stride or get in the way of your arm and pole swing.

Footwear

Your feet will be doing a lot of work when Nordic walking so consider a sock with good cushioning, especially around the heel and on the ball of your foot. The active heel/toe roll coupled with a probable increase in speed means your feet are likely to get hot and sweaty, so choose a sock with good wicking ability and odour-management qualities. Avoid cotton socks and ones that bunch up round your toes or have rough seams that will irritate your feet.

For Nordic walking you want outer footwear that fits well and has a flexible sole. This enables you to achieve a proper heel/toe roll, a key part of the technique. Shoes generally have more pliable soles than boots, but boots offer important ankle protection and more support for your foot.

Soggy feet will ruin a good walk. If possible, buy waterproof footwear. Leather and Gore-Tex or similar waterproof membranes allow your foot to breathe while preventing water penetrating. You will need to re-waterproof boots and shoes regularly if you want them to stay in good condition. If your footwear isn't waterproof, a great alternative is to buy some waterproof socks.

As every foot is different, there is no one perfect shoe. Try before you buy and opt for something that's reasonably light. If your footwear is too heavy, you will end your walk with tight or sore hip flexors. I've tried dozens of shoes and boots over the years and generally wear a Gore-Tex shoe in the summer months and a leather boot through the winter. One of the most popular boots among my clients is the Scarpa Terra GTX, which has a leather outer, good ankle support and a flexible sole.

EIGHT

Exercise Intensity And Goals

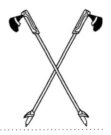

Physical fitness isn't just about your aerobic fitness, although that is a key indicator. It also includes your strength, endurance, flexibility and things like your co-ordination, balance, speed, power, agility and reaction time.

Recommended exercise levels

You should take into account the current health guidelines for adults and older adults.[49] As you get older, things like balance and flexibility typically decrease, so you need to make sure that you are building activities that protect and improve these things into your life. The UK Chief Medical Officers recommend the following:

For those aged nineteen to sixty-four:

- Aim to be physically active every day.

- Develop or maintain strength of muscles by doing heavy gardening, carrying heavy shopping or resistance exercise two days a week.

- At least 150 minutes of activity, such as brisk walking or cycling, or 75 minutes of vigorous activity like running, each week, or even shorter durations of high-intensity activity such as sprinting, stair climbing, or a combination.

- Minimise time spent being sedentary and break up long periods of inactivity.

For the over-sixty-fives:

- Some physical activity is better than none.

- Do some activity to improve muscle strength, balance and flexibility twice a week.

- Each week, do 150 minutes of moderate-intensity aerobic activity, building up gradually, or (if already active) 75 minutes of vigorous activity, or a combination.

- Break up prolonged periods of being sedentary with light activity when possible, with standing at the least.

Nordic walking can go a long way toward meeting these health guidelines. With the correct technique, you will work all your main muscle groups and maintain or even improve the range of motion in your shoulders and general flexibility. Nordic walking helps improve balance and, for most of us, it will be a moderate to vigorous intensity aerobic activity, depending on how we use it. Even so, you can supplement your Nordic walking with additional stretches and resistance work using exercise bands or weights to ensure you meet all of your physical fitness needs.

Exercise intensity

To get the most from your Nordic walks, you need to know how hard you are working. That is, how hard your heart and lungs are having to work to pump the blood around your body. Exercising at the right intensity will prevent you from exercising too hard or not hard enough. Exercise intensity can be roughly split into three broad bands:

Low intensity. This is the ideal level for the beginning and end of a walk, as it helps to improve blood flow and circulation to your working muscles. You are unlikely to be working hard enough to improve your aerobic fitness. It's why ambling round the shops all day won't make you any fitter.

Moderate intensity. Great for developing endurance and burning calories. Due to energy demands, training in this intensity zone will cause your body to utilise both carbs and fats for energy. This makes it great for weight loss and building general fitness.

High intensity. You will only be able to work at this level for a short period of time. It takes you out of your comfort zone and improves your body's ability to utilise oxygen. Hills and fast walking may get you to this level. Combining short bursts of high-intensity exercise with moderate or low-intensity walking is a type of HIIT (high-intensity interval training). It is an efficient way to increase your aerobic fitness and burn calories.

Exercise intensity is highly individual. What feels like hard work to you may feel easy (or harder still) to someone else. The fitter you get, the more you will have to push yourself to reach the same intensity level your less-fit self was working at. It's like a game of cat and mouse. Your fitness is constantly catching up with you, so you've got to keep one step ahead.

How hard you're working when exercising can be measured either scientifically, using heart rate monitors, or by way of estimation. Many of us now wear fitness trackers or smart watches, which track our heart and work rate and calculate the intensity of exercise for us. But you can still estimate the intensity without any gadgets. I particularly like something called the Talk Test'.[50] It is easy to use and centred completely around you and how you are feeling on any particular day. It never gives a false reading, nor does it require any gadgets. You just need to be able to talk and breathe, which is generally something most Nordic walkers are good at.

The Talk Test

Intensity	Walking pace on flat ground	Talk test	How does it feel?	Average walking pace
Low	Normal pace	You can walk and talk easily	No change in your heart rate or breathing pattern	3mph/5km/h
Moderate	Brisk pace	You can talk in short sentences/you can talk but can't sing	You need to breathe more deeply and frequently; you can feel your heart working	4mph/6.5km/h
High	Fast pace	You can only talk in snatches/you don't want to talk at all	You need to breathe hard and deep; your heart is thumping in your chest	Over 4mph/6.5km/h

Note that the average walking speeds above are 'rule of thumb' averages when walking on flat ground. With good technique and decent fitness your fast pace could be over 5mph (8km/h), which is typically a running speed. Annoyingly, aerobic capacity decreases with age so you will not be able to walk as fast in your seventies as you could in your forties.

If and when you want to, there are various ways you can increase your exercise intensity when Nordic walking, which can be a very energetic exercise if you wish it to be. Below are a few ways to do this.

Pace walk

A pace walk is where you walk as fast as you can for a short distance or length of time. Not only will this increase your speed, but it is an excellent way to improve your aerobic fitness. In a pace walk, you should be aiming for high intensity (where you can talk in short snatches only – see the Talk Test above). See the menu for speed in chapter nine for more tips on how to walk fast.

Interval walk

An interval walk is where you vary the intensity you are walking at, either by increasing your speed or by adding inclines or steps. This is a form of high-intensity interval training.

The more frequently you inject an interval walk, the harder your workout. Adding both pace and inclines makes it harder still. If you are using speed, alternate between walking fast and walking at a steady pace. Either for a set time, a set number of paces, or by using markers such as lamp posts, benches or trees that you walk fast between. If you are using inclines or steps, walk up as fast as you can, keeping a steady pace. You can repeat several times, using the return as your recovery. This is my favourite way of turning walking into a high-cardio exercise.

There is increasing evidence to suggest that a HIIT workout can produce health benefits comparable to twice as much moderate-intensity exercise and it is excellent for burning calories quickly. It allows your heart and muscles to go through alternating cycles of work and rest, making them more robust and building strength.

Carrying more load

It takes more effort – and therefore more calories – to move a heavier you, so consider taking a weighted (or filled) backpack on your walk. Be careful with how you carry extra weight; centre it close to your body using a well-fitting backpack.

Different terrain

One way to increase or vary the intensity of your walking, is to walk over different terrains. Love them or hate them, slopes and hills are a feature of much of the UK. Aside from the fact that there's generally a great view to be had at the top, incorporating slopes and hills increases the intensity of any walk. Your heart and lungs work harder, you burn more calories, and you increase the workout for your muscles. When you walk up a hill, do so at a steady pace. It's better to walk at a continuous, if slower, pace than start off fast and have to stop halfway up.

If you don't usually enjoy walking up or down hills, you will love the difference Nordic walking makes. Uphill, it's much easier with poles; downhill, the Nordic walking technique helps protect your knees and hips and gives you greater stability.

Walking uphill

A lot of people fold themselves forward to get up a hill, using their lower back muscles to help haul them up the slope. This places a lot of pressure on muscles that weren't designed for that sort of job, leaving you vulnerable to back ache. It's natural to lean into a slope but the lean should be from your ankle, not at your hip crease. Imagine someone's winching you up from your chest, like a boat being pulled up a ramp out of the water. You'll find that your stride will generally increase on gentle slopes and shorten on steeper inclines. Remember that your leg muscles and glutes are the powerhouse you need for hills and with Nordic walking your upper body contributes too, so it's important not to tighten up your arm swing. Below are some further tips on how to Nordic walk uphill safely:

Top tips

- **Keep your head lifted** (unless the ground is uneven or rocky, in which case safety trumps posture). If your head drops it will pull the rest of your body out of alignment, which will make walking uphill harder.

- **Relax your neck and shoulders.**

- **Drive through your hip** as you push off with your toes and actively use all your leg muscles.

- **Keep a full arm swing for as long as you can.** Reaching forward so that your poles grab the ground ahead of you is like going up a hill in four-wheel drive.

- **Extend the push behind you and rotate**; this will give you extra power.

- **Heel/toe roll for as long as feels comfortable**, then move to a mid-foot to toe motion and only go onto your tiptoes when absolutely necessary. By continuing to heel/toe roll you will stretch and work your calf, lessening the intensity of the workout in that muscle and allowing the muscles above it (your hamstrings and glutes) to activate properly.

- **Walk at a comfortable, steady pace.** This enables your body to get into a rhythm and optimise energy expenditure.

- **Double-arm poling is useful going uphill.**

Common mistakes

- *Ø* **Bending over at the waist.**

- *Ø* **Dropping your head and looking down.**

- *Ø* **Walking on tiptoe.**

- *Ø* **Shortening your arm swing** or clamping your upper arm to the side of your body.

- *Ø* **Stop/starting.** If you watch experienced walkers, you will see that they maintain a steady pace the whole way up a hill. Assess the hill, recognise your fitness level and start at a pace you can sustain.

Walking downhill

Many people are anxious about walking downhill, especially when the ground is stony or slippy. It is sensible to be cautious going down slopes, especially rocky ones. It is de-stabilising and may cause your knees to ache or bring back memories of having fallen over before. Happily, there are some helpful tips for downhill walking, many of which are relevant even if you don't have your Nordic walking poles with you:

Top tips

- *Ø* **Soften your knees and drop your centre of gravity** to just behind your knee-caps so that your weight is between your heel and the middle of your foot. This will take the pressure off your knees and toes. The steeper the slope, the more you will need to bend your knees.

- **Shorten your stride**; you will feel more stable and in control.

- **Tuck your tailbone under you.**

- **Tighten your glutes** if possible (it takes practice). This 'glues' you to the ground.

- **Keep your head up** where possible and your chest lifted; relax your neck and shoulders.

- **Push through your hip** – this will help you go downhill faster while maintaining good balance.

- **Keep the poles angled backward** and maintain strong downward pressure; this will help anchor you, giving you great stability.

- **Consider zigzagging downhill** if there's space to do so.

- **On a very steep slope, or if you're nervous, place the poles in front** and use them as brakes.

- **Unclip your straps from the pole** if you are worried about falling and want your hands to be free.

Common mistakes

- **Leaning forward down the slope.** This is a very unstable position and puts a lot of stress on your joints.

- **Propelling yourself forward with your poles.** Again, this will destabilise you.

Muddy ground

There's little chance of avoiding muddy ground if you want to walk off-road year-round in the UK. Fortunately, Nordic walking poles provide valuable support on slippy surfaces and, in many ways, walking on mud gives you a great workout. Your legs work harder, both getting through the mud and stopping you from sliding sideways in it. Your stomach muscles engage to help you keep your balance and stop you slipping backwards, and your upper body and arms are needed to help you stabilise through your poles. This means you'll be burning plenty of calories and toning your whole body. It's important to ensure you stretch properly at the end of a muddy walk as stabilising your body puts a lot of strain on your hips and legs. In addition, follow the tips below for muddy Nordic walking:

Top tips

- **Push the pole firmly into the ground** to stop you skidding around and maintain downward pressure through the pole for continued support.

- **Relax your neck and shoulders** and draw your belly toward your spine to engage your core muscles and give you greater balance.

- **Reduce your arm swing.** You want your poles to stay close to your body to give support.

- **Wear gaiters** to protect your trousers.

Common mistakes

- **Wearing wellies/the wrong footwear.** Nordic walking in wellies doesn't work unless your wellies are well fitted and give your foot good support. You shouldn't have any lumps of mud stuck to the base of your boots after a muddy walk. If you do, your footwear isn't appropriate.

- **Lifting and tensing your shoulders.**

- **Over-striding**; try to keep your stride short when on slippery ground.

- **Double-arm poling.**

Pavements or hard ground

At some stage, you will probably be walking on pavements, tarmac or similar hard ground. Walking on this type of surface is, in many ways, excellent. It's far less forgiving than grass so you can hear whether your rhythm is even and correct it if not. It also provides a good workout for the muscles around your middle, which help with stability and balance.

On the downside, walking on hard surfaces increases the stresses on your body, especially your tibia (shin bone), and can result in shin splints. This isn't an issue if you are only doing short bursts but if you're regularly pavement walking, it's advisable to buy some training shoes with good shock absorption. Walking boots and shoes aren't designed for this type of surface and generally won't provide sufficient cushioning. Walking on hard surfaces also increases the vibration through your Nordic walking poles, which can feel uncomfortable.

Almost all Nordic walking poles are sold with 'paws'. These are rubber stoppers that cover the metal tip at the base of the pole. Most people use the paws when walking on tarmac or similar hard ground in the belief that it's quieter and that the tips may be damaged if they're not protected. Neither of these points is strictly true. Some tips, such as the Exel racing spike, which has its own inbuilt suspension system, are as quiet as most paws. Also, the tips are made of tungsten carbide, an extremely strong metal, so you will not damage them if you use them uncovered. The only potential problem is that, very occasionally, the metal tip might remain embedded in the tarmac, although this generally only happens if it was faulty and not fixed properly when manufactured. So it isn't necessary to cover the metal tip when you walk on tarmac, although you can if you want to. For health and safety reasons it is wise to use paws if you are on a busy pavement.

There's a definite knack to Nordic walking on hard ground and a common problem is that the poles frequently slide, making it difficult to get a good grip and a satisfactory action. Below are some pointers that should help:

Top tips

- **Keep your poles a little more upright than normal** so that the paw makes a good connection with the tarmac.

- **Keep your neck and shoulders relaxed.**

- **Don't extend your arm push** behind your body as the pole will generally start to slide.

- **Use quality Nordic walking poles** with high carbon content to absorb the additional vibration up the pole shaft from walking on a hard surface.

- **The paws will slide** if you hit a patch of loose gravel so avoid these areas if possible.

Common mistakes

- **Pushing the pole fully behind you** – it will just slip.

- **Not pushing down firmly enough.** You need to push through the pole more firmly than you might when walking on grass or a soft surface. This may seem counter intuitive but it gives you a better connection with the walking surface and if you don't the pole will slip. It's why walking on pavements is such a great waist workout, as the harder you push through the pole the more your abdominal muscles engage and strengthen.

- **Wearing the wrong footwear.** You want something with good shock absorption, like trainers.

Goal setting

For some people, goal setting helps motivate them. Even if you don't want to be ruled by achievement targets, I would say that we all have goals, whether that's simply trying to stay generally active or something more tangible, like training for a specific event or losing a set amount of weight.

Goals don't have to be big, just something by which you can measure your progress and give yourself a metaphorical pat on the back. If you're not sure you've got a goal, think about why you picked up this book. Was it because you want to lose weight, resolve a bad back, support rehabilitation from an injury or surgery, walk longer and with less pain, reduce your medication, prepare for a walking holiday or challenge? Have a think and write some things down to refer back to. It may surprise you how quickly you reach them, especially if you establish a regular Nordic walking routine.

For many of my clients, it's the little things that make a big difference when it comes to setting fitness goals and measuring progress. Here's a list of some common ones:

- Progressing from walking on the flat to taking in slopes.

- Clocking how puffed out they feel on a particular hill and assessing their fitness progress each time they go up that hill.

- Doing a particular stretch at the end of their walk and noting how their flexibility increases over the weeks.

- Walking with family or friends and instead of trailing at the back, walking comfortably at the front (if you start Nordic walking regularly, this will happen to you).

- Walking a set route and beating your previous times.

- Nordic walking at a local Park Run (they welcome Nordic walkers) and beating your previous times.

Warm-ups and stretches

In certain cultures many people follow an exercise routine every morning. Squats, arm circles, single leg balance, bending, stretching and jumping are all a standard part of their day. This is not something that we've integrated into our Western culture to the same extent, but a pre-walk mobilisation/muscle activation routine can make a real difference to how much you get out of your Nordic walking. In this section, I share with you my ten favourite warm-ups and stretches. I've used them time and again in all my classes and they deliver every time.

Top ten walking warm-ups

I know that walking is often used as a warm-up in its own right but if you've been sitting down all day, or your body is feeling stiff and a bit static, mobilising your joints and finding some alignment before you head off will help you get the most from your Nordic walk. As Nordic walking uses muscles throughout your body, your whole body will benefit from warm-ups, so let's start from the top:

1. Chin slides

Stand tall, shoulders rolled back and down. Jut your chin forward then slide it backward to bring your earlobes over (or toward) your shoulders, giving yourself a double chin. Don't look down. Keep your chin level to the ground. Repeat six times.

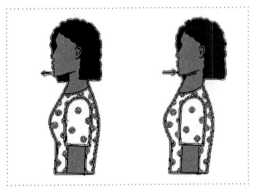

2. Sky reaches

Now we move down with two exercises for the upper body, the first of which is sky reaches. Stand tall, feet wide apart, tummy muscles gently engaged. Hold your poles horizontally above your head, hands wide. Reach your left arm up high, over your head, twisting your body gently and pointing your left toe. Now do the other side. Repeat six times.

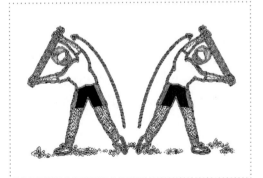

3. Shoulder rolls

Stand tall, feet comfortably apart, tummy muscles gently engaged. Lift your shoulders high toward your ears, then slowly roll them back and down. Repeat six times.

4. Open/close

Turning now to your back and spine, stand tall, feet comfortably apart, shoulders rolled back and down. Open your arms wide, squeezing your shoulder blades together, then round your arms forward like you're hugging a big ball, pulling your shoulder blades apart. Repeat six times. This wakes up the muscles your mid-back area, which are often switched off.

5. Kayaking

Stand tall, feet comfortably apart. Hold your poles horizontally in front with your hands wide. Push one hand up and away from your body and at the same time pull the other hand down and towards your waist. Repeat on the other side. The action is like paddling (or kayaking) down a river. Repeat six times, building up a gentle rhythm.

6. Pelvic rocks

Stand tall, shoulders rolled back and down, feet comfortably apart. Tilt your bottom back as far as it will go. Then tuck it under you, again as far as you can, and pull your pubic bone up toward your ribs. Don't round your upper body, this is an isolated exercise that will help mobilise your lower back, which is very stiff for many people. Repeat six times.

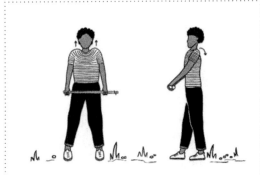

Shoulder rolls

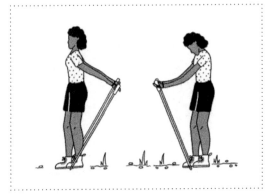

Open/close

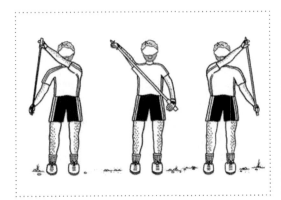

Kayaking

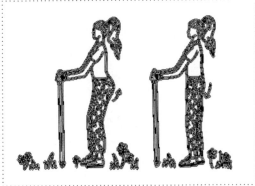

Pelvic rocks

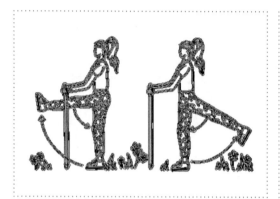

Leg swings

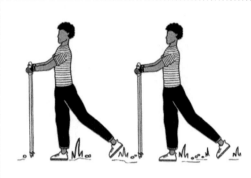

Rear toe taps

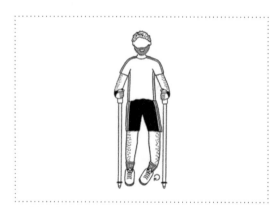

Ankle circles

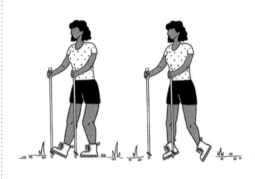

Heel/toe roll

7. Leg swings

Now we move on to your lower body, starting with leg swings from front to back. Repeat six times on each leg.

8. Rear toe taps

These will wake your glutes up. Stand tall, feet comfortably apart. Keep your tailbone tucked under and gently engage your tummy muscles. Put one foot behind you and pulse it up and down, toes pointing to the ground. You should feel this in your buttock. Change legs. Repeat six times on each leg.

9. Ankle circles

Put one foot in front of you. Slowly circle it one way then the other, like you're trying to paint a large circle with your toes. Change legs and repeat six times on each leg.

10. Heel/toe roll

This is most effective if you do both feet together, but it's fine to do one foot at a time. Stand tall, feet comfortably apart. Rock back onto your heels so your toes come up a little, then roll through your foot rising up onto your toes and back down again to your heels. Repeat six times. Don't forget to change sides if you are doing one foot at a time.

Top ten stretches

Doing a few stretches at the end of your walk puts the finishing touches to your walk so that you fully reap the benefits. Rounding off your walk with stretches will improve your flexibility and re-balance your muscles and body.

1. Yes, no, maybe

Again, we'll start at the head. I'm cheating a bit here, as this is actually three separate stretches.

a) Stand tall with your feet comfortably apart, shoulders rolled back and down, tailbone tucked under. First, nod your head slowly backward then forward in a 'yes' gesture. You should feel the stretch at the front and base of your neck. Repeat six times.

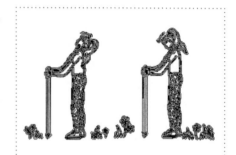

b) Next, slowly turn your head side to side in a 'no' gesture. You should feel the stretch down the side of your neck. Repeat six times.

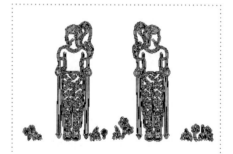

c) Finally, drop one ear down toward your shoulder in a 'maybe' gesture, then return to the centre and drop your other ear down to your other shoulder. Repeat six times.

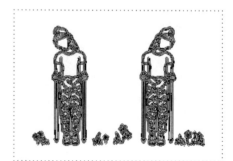

2. Shoulder stretch

Moving down to your upper body, start with a shoulder stretch. Stand tall, feet comfortably apart. Put one arm straight out in front of you, shoulder down. Hook your other arm underneath, just above your elbow, and pull it across. You should feel the stretch in your shoulder muscle. Hold for four breaths. Switch sides and repeat.

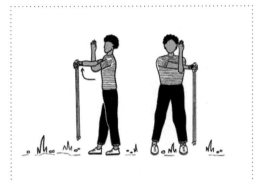

3. Side bend

Stand tall, feet comfortably apart. Hold your poles horizontally above your head, hands wide. Reach up high with one arm and lengthen up and over as you bend to the side. Imagine standing between two panes of glass. You should feel the stretch down your side. Hold for four breaths. Switch sides and repeat.

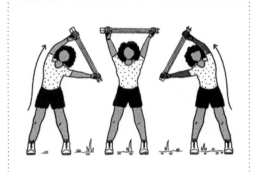

4. Chest stretch

Stand tall, feet comfortably apart. Place the poles horizontally behind your hips with your palms facing backward. Gently lift the poles behind your body keeping your arms straight, your head up and your tailbone tucked under. Hold for four breaths.

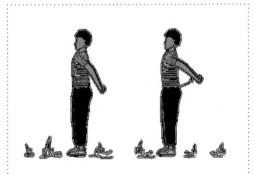

5. Back stretch

Stand with your feet comfortably apart and your poles in front of your body. Walk your feet backwards, dropping your head and bending from your waist until you have a flat back. Take an in breath, then tuck your tailbone under and arch your back upward as you exhale. Return to a flat back and repeat four times in time with your breathing. Feel the stretch in your back.

6. Back extension

Stand tall, feet comfortably apart. Raise the poles horizontally above your head, hands wide. Gently lean your upper body back. Hold for four breaths.

7. Hip and front of thigh

Moving down to your lower body, start with this stretch for your hips and front of thighs. Stand tall, feet comfortably apart. Take one long step backward, with the ball of your back foot on the ground, heel raised. Bend your knees and slowly sink your back knee down toward the ground, like a deep lunge. Keep your body upright. Tuck your tailbone under to increase the stretch. You should feel the stretch in the front of your thigh all the way up to your hip. Hold for four breaths. Switch sides and repeat.

8. Calf and back of thigh

Stand tall, feet comfortably apart. Extend one leg forward, resting on your heel with your toes pointing up. Bend your supporting leg and sit back on it, pushing your chest forward. You should feel the stretch up the back of your straight leg. The closer you pull your toes toward you, the greater the stretch. Hold for four breaths. Switch sides and repeat.

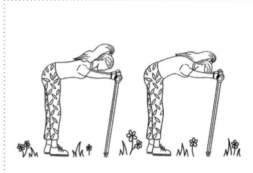

Back stretch

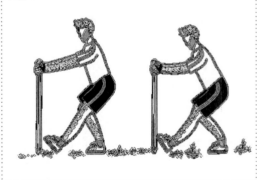

Back extension

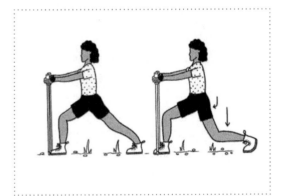

Hip and front thigh

Calf and back of thigh

9. Inner thigh

Stand with your feet wide apart, toes pointing forward. Turn your right foot out slightly and bend your right knee until you feel a stretch in your left inner thigh. Hold for four breaths. Switch sides and repeat.

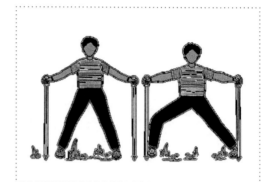

10. Glutes

Stand tall, feet comfortably apart. Place one ankle on top of the opposite thigh, knee out to the side. Bend your supporting knee and hinge forward from your hips. Keep your supporting knee in line with your ankle. You should feel the stretch in your buttock. Hold for four breaths. Switch sides and repeat.

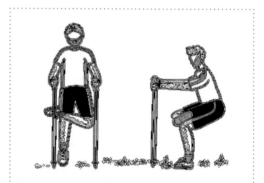

SUMMARY OF PART THREE

At this point in the book, you should know how to choose the right Nordic walking poles for you and what clothing and shoes will help you get the most from your Nordic walking. You should be familiar with the health and fitness recommendations for your age group and have some tools to help you measure and adapt your exercise intensity, set goals and generally stay fit and strong. You know how to walk safely over different terrains, including hills and slopes, and have a variety of warm-ups and stretches you can use to increase your strength, flexibility and whole-body benefits.

PART FOUR

NORDIC WALKING MENUS

In this part of the book, we're going to talk about fitness, wellbeing, looking after your body and health conditions. Each chapter contains a brief introduction, warm-up exercises, top tips and common mistakes related to these four topics, all based on the Four Steps to Success I introduced earlier. The Four Steps are your tools and here I will explain exactly how to use them to maximise your benefits.

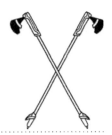

NINE

Fitness Menus

In this chapter, I provide you with four Nordic walking fitness menus focusing on speed, weight loss, muscle tone and distance walking, respectively. They are designed to give you targeted support if you are using Nordic walking as an alternative to running, as part of a cross-training or weight loss programme, or to prepare for a challenge event or hike. We'll start with speed and how Nordic walking can help you to walk faster.

Speed

Nordic walking is the ultimate way to increase your walking speed as the pole design and technique are both geared toward propelling you forward faster than you would normally be able to do. None of my clients have ever gone slower with a pair of poles in their hands unless it was deliberate, for example on a mindfulness walk.

As well as covering more distance in less time, increasing your walking speed raises your heart rate further, increases your aerobic fitness and burns more calories. Nordic walking is therefore an ideal exercise if you are transitioning from running to walking and want to achieve a similar level of intensity.

Walking at a fast pace doesn't need to be maintained for a long time to be effective. Bursts of faster walking can be built into your regular walk to up the intensity. The longer you walk at a fast pace, the fitter you will get. Walking fast requires excellent posture, a good walking action and the Nordic walking technique. It's not easy to do as a beginner, so I suggest you start with short periods of fast walking and gradually build it up.

The best exercises for increasing speed are:

- Kayaking
- Rear toe taps
- Heel/toe roll

Top tips

- **Arms, legs, feet.** These are your three speed accelerators; the quicker you move them the faster you'll go.

- **Posture.** The faster you walk, the harder it will be to maintain good posture, but it is essential to keep your bones and joints in alignment. Good alignment will allow your muscles to work more efficiently and decrease stress on your body (and the potential for injury). Set your posture before you start walking at speed and keep coming back to it, focusing in particular on releasing tension in your neck and shoulders as these often tighten when walking fast.

- **Establish your breathing rhythm.** You don't want to out-walk your breath. Sync your breathing with your steps. The faster you walk, the harder it will be to breathe in through your nose, due to your body's increased need for oxygen, but you can train yourself to breathe this way even at fast speeds.

Work your feet. Increase the speed of your heel/toe roll and you will walk faster. Keep your action smooth and accurate. Let gravity pull you forward; this will give you more momentum and help you go faster.

Make your glutes a powerhouse. Ensure you are squeezing your glutes, that powerful trio of muscles in your buttocks, when you push off with your toes. They were designed for speed and will make you go faster.

Quicken your steps (cadence). The faster you move your legs, the more steps per minute you'll take. As a rule of thumb, over 100 steps per minute is a brisk walking pace for most people. When you reach a pace of 140 steps per minute you should be on the verge of jogging.

Clean, fast pole placement. Place your pole in the ground right at the point your arm starts its backward swing. Lots of people miss out on extra power and speed because they've not got their pole in the ground or applied downward pressure fast enough.

Speed up your arm swing. Push back quickly and smoothly, keeping the pole pressed down into the ground with a good amount of force for as long as possible. Your arm swing must keep pace with your legs, so you might not be able to extend your arm swing far behind your body if you are walking fast.

Rotate your upper body. Like a coiled spring unwinding, the natural rotation of your torso will increase your speed.

Relax. Keep your neck and shoulders soft. Don't be rigid. Let it flow and you'll fly.

Common mistakes

- **Forcing your stride length.** Don't reach out farther with your foot to increase your stride length as it won't make you go faster. In fact, it's likely to have the opposite effect, acting as a break and potentially also jarring your back and knees. Instead, increase your leg push behind you.

- **Bouncing.** Bobbing up and down wastes time and energy. If you want to go fast, aim to glide across the ground like a swan glides across the water, with your head and neck relaxed and 'floating' above the powerhouse of the rest of your body.

- **Lifting your shoulders.** Be careful that your shoulders don't rise and tense up.

- **Not stretching post-walk.** To avoid injury and re-balance your muscles, you need to stretch.

How to use BPM to increase and maintain your walking pace

The number of steps you take per minute is called your cadence. A great way to increase and maintain your cadence is to walk to the beat of music or use a metronome. Our bodies like to walk to a rhythm or beat, so walking to music with a BPM (beats per minute) that correlates to your target walking pace will help you reach and maintain that pace. Plus, you're less likely to slow down if you get distracted or lost in your thoughts, or when you start to feel tired. The faster the beat, the quicker your pace.

There are apps and programmes that can help you put together playlists with a certain BPM or you can simply type your desired BPM into the search bar of your music player and it will produce a list.

An alternative to listening to music is to download a metronome app on your smartphone or use a portable digital metronome. I've started using one recently with great results. I simply set the metronome to my goal BPM, clip it to my waistbelt and off I go. I can increase and decrease the BPM by simply pressing the plus and minus buttons, so it's more versatile than having to change music tracks.

The ideal BPM to walk to will vary from person to person. Research suggests that over 100 steps per minute (2.7mph) qualifies as a brisk walking pace for many people.[51] My cadence for fast walking is around 140bpm. Once I go above this, my technique suffers and by 150bpm I'm wanting to start running.

While all of these tips will help you speed up, if you want to increase your exercise intensity this way, you don't need to walk fast to get results from Nordic walking and in fact a slower walk is better for upper body muscle tone. But knowing how to Nordic walk fast is great in a challenge event, if you want to boost your cardiovascular benefits, lose weight, or simply if you want to get places quicker.

Weight loss

Nordic walking is energy thirsty. As mentioned previously, with good technique, you can use up to 46% more calories Nordic walking than regular walking.[52] This is not only because the Nordic walking action propels you to walk faster, but also because of how many more muscles it brings into play – your arms, shoulders, upper body and increased core work. This extra muscle requirement demands more energy and burns more calories.

Another benefit is that although Nordic walking is more intense than regular walking, it doesn't feel like it because the workload is spread across your body and the poles act as support. This makes losing weight easier and, best of all, you can talk at the same time.

Whether you exercise regularly or are new to it, to lose weight through Nordic walking you need to manipulate the following three variables:

- **Duration** – how long you walk for.

- **Intensity** – how hard your body is working. We discussed earlier how to vary the intensity of your walk, but to summarise, you can do this by increasing your walking speed, walking on uneven or unstable surfaces (such as sand or mud), walking up hills, or carrying a weighted backpack.

- **Frequency** – how often you walk.

The key is to mix things up. See my top tips on using Nordic walking to lose weight below. The best exercises to focus on for weight loss are:

- Open/close

- Kayaking

- Rear toe taps

Top tips

- **Maintain good posture** to avoid injury. Bad posture can cause you to lose your momentum and sabotage your weight loss.

- **Use your full technique.** It's easy to switch off from using your whole body and the proper Nordic walking technique, especially when walking fast or for a long time, but using more muscles uses more energy. Check in regularly with your leg muscles, heel/toe roll, glutes, arms and rotation to keep your technique sharp.

- **Mix it up.** Using a mix of long steady paced walks, fast walks and intervals is the best way to lose weight and get fit. Include inclines to make it more challenging still.

- **Schedule your walks.** If you want to prioritise weight loss, scheduling walks into your diary will ensure they're not forgotten and happen regularly.

- **Keep your body guessing.** If you do the same thing over and over again, your body will adapt to the new normal and your weight loss will plateau. Keep things fresh by having two or three different routes, with inclines and new terrains at different points in the walk so that you don't follow the same pattern every time.

- **Use the Talk Test.** (See chapter eight.) Use your breathing to build a steady and comfortable walking rhythm and gauge how hard you are working. To burn calories, you want to be in the 'talk but can't sing' zone. That's the equivalent to the 'fat burn' zone you hear about at the gym. You also burn lots of calories when you are working at the harder 'talk in short sentences only/don't want to talk at all' level, but this is difficult to sustain for long, so use this for your interval and pace sessions. If you are walking and talking comfortably you won't be burning many calories. Avoid spending too much time in this zone. Fitness apps and heart rate monitors are widely used and are a helpful way of monitoring your exercise intensity.

- **Long walks = weight loss.** Do at least one long steady paced (talk but can't sing) walk a week and aim to increase how long you walk for each week. See the section on endurance walks later in this chapter for some technique tips for long walks.

- **Walk in the morning.** Research suggests that morning exercise is best for weight loss, especially for women.[53] Walking in the morning also ensures your exercise is done before life gets in the way.

- **Make yourself accountable.** Walking with a friend, joining a Nordic walking group, using a fitness app or any other way of making yourself accountable to others will help keep you focused and engaged. It's fun too.

- **Sign up for a challenge.** One of the best ways to stay motivated is to sign up for a walking challenge. This gives you a deadline to work toward. All walking challenges I've come across permit Nordic walking and many running challenges do too, although they generally ask you to start at the back so you don't trip anyone up.

Common mistakes

- **'Treating' yourself to a high-calorie drink or food** after you've been out Nordic walking. If you're walking to burn calories and lose weight, this will undo your hard work. Plan ahead and take something nutritious with you instead.

- **Doing too much too soon**, especially if you haven't exercised for a while. This will risk injury. Gradually build up the number of walks you do and the duration/distance.

- **Not stretching afterward.** Plantar fasciitis (where you get pain in the bottom of your foot) is a particular problem for walkers. The main cure is rest so it would derail any weight loss goals if you were to develop this. Stretching your leg muscles and rolling your foot over a tennis or spiky ball daily will help prevent it.

If you are new to exercise, how often you walk is more important than how hard or for how long you walk. By simply establishing a consistent habit of three or more walks each week, you can achieve astonishing results.

Tone, trim and strengthen

Nordic walking is a muscle toning and strengthening exercise and a great alternative to the gym. You can work all your main muscle groups while chatting and even walking your dog. It almost sounds too good to be true, but that's because we have been conditioned to think we have to do something over and above the ordinary to achieve fitness results. This isn't true. Gyms and personal trainers barely existed fifty years ago and people were just as strong then as they are now – maybe even more so, because they led more active lives.

Nordic walking is the outdoor equivalent of a cross-trainer. With the correct technique you can streamline your hips and thighs, trim your waist, tone the backs of your arms and sculpt your shoulders. It targets your whole body. You don't have to lose weight to lose inches and you don't have to go to the gym to strengthen your muscles.

These exercises and warm-ups will wake up your waist, warm up your shoulders and fire up your glutes so that you can get maximum muscle toning benefits from Nordic walking:

- Sky reaches
- Kayaking
- Leg swings
- Rear toe taps
- Heel/toe roll

Top tips

- **By lengthening your spine and lifting your chest** up and away from your hips, you will instantly feel (and look) slimmer.

- **Gently pull your tummy button in** toward your spine, maintain downward pressure through your pole as you push it back and rotate your upper body. This will strengthen your middle and trim your waist. I've found that walking on tarmac or other hard surfaces increases my waist workout.

- **Extend your arm swing.** Nordic walking is amazing for your upper arms and shoulders and, if you walk often enough with good technique, you can sculpt both. The fuller your arm swing, the greater your arm tone, so extend your backswing behind your hip if you can. It takes time to build enough arm strength to do this. Single-arm poling (using just one pole while carrying the other) and double-arm poling (both arms together) are both excellent for arm and shoulder tone.

- **Include hills.** You'll work your thighs, backs of legs and buttocks even harder when going up hills. Maintain your heel/toe action for as long as feels comfortable to achieve maximum benefit and don't bend over at your waist. Check back to the hills section in chapter eight.

- **Vary your speed.** By slowing your pace you can keep your pole in the ground for longer, giving you the opportunity to increase your chest, waist and arm workout. If you walk fast, your legs will benefit more.

- **Reduce your body fat.** Fat obscures the definition of muscle so if you want to see increased muscle tone, you will need to decrease your body fat. Muscle uses more energy (calories) and increasing your muscle tone will increase the number of calories your body needs. Muscle is also heavier than fat so your weight may not reduce even though your trouser size does.

- **Add lunges and other exercises.** Adding a few walking lunges or squats will strengthen and tone your legs more quickly, while stopping at benches and doing push-ups or bench dips will benefit your arms, shoulders and chest.

- **Stretch afterward.** Stretching returns balance to your muscles and body. If you don't stretch regularly, you will be more prone to injury.

Common mistakes

- **Dropping your chest.** You won't whittle your waist or strengthen your pecs if your chest is slumped. Firm downward pressure through your pole perks up your pecs and lifts a sagging chest.

- **Rounding or lifting your shoulders.** To get the most out of Nordic walking, you need to walk with your shoulders wide and down.

- **Missing your pole placement at the front.** To increase the arm swing behind their body it's common for Nordic walkers to shorten the front part of their swing. This is usually because their arms aren't yet strong enough for the full action. However, you will miss out on power and arm tone by shortening your arm action at the front, so keep a strong forward swing.

- **Lazy feet.** 'Buns of steel' are all about strong glutes. A powerful push off with your toes will fire these up and help create a pert bottom. Focus on your heel/toe roll and actively squeeze your buttock as you toe-off. You'll know you're doing it right when you can feel the muscles up the back of your legs tightening and your buttocks squeezing. You'll need shoes with a flexible sole to maximise the benefits.

Although Nordic walking uses your whole body, I still recommend that clients incorporate additional exercises like lunges, squats, push-ups and shoulder presses a couple of times a week. These can be tagged on to your Nordic walk. Maintaining muscle strength is crucial for healthy bones, balance and reducing the risk of injury.

Endurance walking

Signing up for an endurance or challenge walk is what triggers many people to start using poles. Usually they buy trekking poles, but Nordic walking has so much more to offer. I explained in detail the differences between Nordic walking and trekking in chapter one, but to recap, switching to Nordic walking when taking on a challenge or endurance walk will benefit your posture, walking action and speed. This means a more enjoyable walk, fewer aches afterwards and a quicker time.

Nordic walking has made the world of difference in the many challenges I've done. Particular standouts were completing four marathons in four days along the hilly Cotswold Way, where I had not a single blister while the feet of other participants were in shreds; a 10km road race where I overtook dozens of joggers; and a fifty-two-mile Sense Charity walk, where my trusty Nordic walking poles and technique carried me through the day/night challenge, again with no blisters.

If you are an endurance runner or triathlete, I would urge you to consider incorporating Nordic walking into your training schedule. The poles will take pressure off your joints and the technique will help you stay injury-free, plus Nordic walking poles double up as trail running poles, so you can walk/run in combination.

The best exercises if you're using Nordic walking to train for a challenge or endurance event are:

- Chin slides
- Shoulder rolls
- Open/close
- Pelvic rocks
- Leg swings
- Ankle circles

Top tips

- **Frequently do a body-scan to check your posture.** Correct alignment becomes increasingly important the longer you're walking for. If your feet are working properly and your body is correctly stacked over your bones, muscles, ligaments and fascia, everything will work harmoniously and you will optimise your efficiency. I use the acronym SHREK as my reminder: shoulders (rolled back and down, level), hips (level), ribs (lifted), ears (stacked over shoulders), knees (facing forward, weight evenly distributed).

- **Keep your breathing steady.** Starting and stopping takes more muscular effort and energy than sustained walking at a steady pace, so try not to let yourself get out of breath or stop/start, especially when going up hills.

- **Fully extend your leg behind you** so that your knee is straight when you push off; this will engage your powerful glutes and open the front part of your hips. Tight hips are common on a long walk and this will prevent them from getting stiff and sore.

- **Use your circulation pumps.** Lifting your toes for your heel strike and squeezing your hand round the pole handle both help to pump the blood back up through your veins to your heart. This is useful on a long walk, especially on a hot day, and will stop your feet, legs and hands puffing up.

- **Regulate your arm push power.** One of the beautiful things about Nordic walking is that your arms and shoulders are part of your walking action, but be careful not to overdo it on a long walk and end up with arm fatigue. This could cause you to adapt your arm swing, which would typically manifest as hinging at your elbow, causing aching in that delicate elbow joint.

- **Consider replacing Nordic walking straps with gloves.** Leki and a few other pole manufacturers sell strap-integrated Nordic walking gloves. They are highly breathable, come in short- and long-fingered styles and help distribute the load over your hand as you push through the strap. These are especially useful on a long walk.

- **Trim your toenails.** Clipping your toenails before a long walk will help prevent bruised, sore toes. It's so simple, yet often overlooked.

- **Wear good shoes with flexible soles.** Well-fitting shoes or boots with room for your toes to expand are a must. No matter how good your body feels, if your feet are sore and blistering, your walk is ruined. Consider also lacing your boots differently, especially if your toes tend to jam against the front of your toe-box on steep downhill sections. There's a surprising number of different lacing techniques, including one that gives a better heel hold.

- **Take a second pair of socks.** We have 250,000 sweat glands in our feet, which can produce up to half a pint of perspiration daily.[54] Having the correct socks is therefore as important as having the correct shoes on a long walk and changing them part way through will refresh your feet and help prevent blisters.

🌿 **Choose a well-fitting backpack.** There are hundreds of daypack styles to choose from, but a chest strap is essential as it ensures your pack sits snugly. I also value a hip belt, which takes the pack weight off my shoulders.

Common mistakes

🌿 **Doing too much too soon.** Just like training for a marathon, you need to build up your fitness, strength and stamina for a long walk.

🌿 **Slumping and poor technique when you start to tire.** It's tempting to bend over at your waist, shorten your gait and walk flat-footed when you get tired, but you will lose efficiency and rely on muscles that weren't designed for the job.

🌿 **Too much wrist flexion/extension.** Nordic walking requires a firm wrist; if you have too much movement in your wrist, it will get very sore over a long walk.

Anticipating blisters

You want to do all you can to avoid getting blisters. They're painful and can spoil your day as well as your walk. Take blister plasters and apply as soon as you feel a hot spot developing. Ideally, do your utmost to not get them in the first place, which means:

🌿 Properly fitting walking boots/shoes.

🌿 Good socks – ones without rough seams and which wick the moisture away.

- Taping up any worry areas with microporous (or similar) blue physio tape in advance of walking. Or you could consider wrapping sheep's wool around your toes – many of my clients have told me this is amazing for preventing blisters.
- Taking your boots off during breaks and/or changing your socks.

TEN

Wellbeing Menus

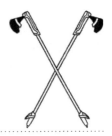

The menus provided in this chapter are centred around wellbeing. Use them to build a practice of Nordic walking for mindfulness and easing stress, regaining your balance and confidence, managing the menopause, strengthening your pelvic floor and to maximise your overall health and wellbeing as an older adult.

Mindfulness

Walking, especially walking in nature, is one of the greatest gifts you can give your mental health. It seems extraordinary that something as simple as going for a walk and taking in the natural beauty around you can have such a positive effect on your mood and sense of wellbeing, but research consistently shows this to be the case. It reduces blood pressure, heart rate, muscle tension, and the stress hormone cortisol. A calm, mindful walk has immense healing power.

There are two different ways to approach a mindful Nordic walk. You can focus inward, on your breathing, the movement of your body, what your feet are doing and your Nordic walking technique. Or, you can shift your attention outward, taking in the natural world around you and connecting with it. Both bring stillness and calm, re-balancing the brain–body relationship.

If you're interested in wildflowers, butterflies and trees, there are some fantastic free smartphone apps that can tell you then and there what you're looking at. All you have to do is upload a photo. See the resources section at the end of the book for more information.

Speed is not your aim on this kind of walk. Your goal is not to rush. Slowing down your walking pace helps slow down your brain, especially beneficial if it feels like it's going a hundred miles an hour. Another good way to switch off an over-active mind is to engage your senses. Your senses bridge the gap between you and the natural world and help give your thoughts a rest. Allow your senses to feel, smell, taste, hear and see as you walk, and your thoughts to drop away.

ENGAGE YOUR SENSES

Feel the air on your body, the breeze on your face and hands. Notice how your clothes press against your skin, the Nordic walking straps on your hands, and how the pole handle moves in your hand as you swing your arms. As you breathe in, what can you smell? It can take a while to tune into this sense. There might be one obvious smell, but can you distinguish other smells and separate them out? Listen to the layers of noise around you, starting with the noise furthest away and finishing with what's closest to you, even the ringing within your ears. Listen to the silence between sounds and how different noises layer with each other like different instruments in an orchestra. Notice the colours around you. The shadows. The movement in the plants. Take in the sky and the clouds, the way they move, shift and re-shape. Engaging your senses in this way will help to take you out of your everyday thoughts and worries and into nature.

Before you embark on your mindfulness walk, do the following exercises:

- Open/close
- Rotate

These will raise your ribs and expand your breathing and soothe your spine, getting you in the best state to embark on a mindful walk. Below are my top tips for turning Nordic walking into a deliberately mindful activity:

Top tips

- **Remove distractions.** Leave behind or switch off your phone, camera, music and other distractions. Instead, connect with your senses, nature and the world around you.

- **Feel your posture.** Take time to enjoy the sensation of your spine lengthening, your head and chest lifting and your ears sliding back over your shoulders. Gently roll your shoulders back and feel the weight of your arms pulling your shoulders down. Sense how these movements realign your body, reducing tension. Soften your scalp, soften your brain. Wiggle your head and jaw and relax your face.

- **Breathing** is one of the easiest ways to clear your mind, relax your body and bring yourself back into the present moment. Use the technique set out in the second part of this book to breathe down and wide. Syncing your steps with your breathing is a well-known mindfulness technique. Air provides oxygen and energy; pull this in as you inhale. I like to count my steps breathing in and breathing out. Don't force your breath, just count it with your steps. Try to focus on counting and not letting your mind flit to other things. If it does (which is almost inevitable), just bring it back to your breathing and start again.

- **'Ground' yourself** by feeling each footstep: the lifting of your toes toward your knee; the roll of your foot from heel to toes; how your ankle moves; your feet within your shoes and how your weight shifts through your foot with each step; the surface you are walking over. Be aware how shifting your weight forward engages the core muscles and pulls your body forward into the next step. Notice how your core muscles support your back.

- **Use your Nordic walking poles to build a steady rhythm.** Focus your attention on your technique: your arm swing and hand control, the sensation of being propelled forward. Observe your movements.

- **Imagine any tension is like water** and you are draining it down and away through your body (like a sieve). Try doing this in two stages with each out-breath. First, from your head, neck and shoulders to your belly button. Then, from your belly button, down through your legs and feet and away into the ground. You may want to repeat this several times and keep coming back to it throughout your walk.

- **When you finish**, stand somewhere pleasant. Recognise that everything is a cycle. Busy time. Rest. Busy time. Rest.

Common mistakes

- **Chatting the whole way through your walk** when walking with friends. Try being with them but not always talking – for example, five minutes inward focus, five minutes outward focus (engage your senses), five minutes chatting and sharing.

- **Getting distracted.** Often, clients say that focusing on the technique is a form of mindfulness because it's completely absorbing.

🌿 **Getting cross with yourself** for letting your thoughts catch up with you. Accept that they will enter your mind, and just let them pass through.

Exercising mindfully is just like exercise for physical benefit – the more you do, the easier it becomes and the more you will get from it. Just a few minutes finding your calm through walking mindfully will make a difference and you can build it into any walk you do.

Balance and confidence

Somewhere along the way as we age there can be an ebbing away of confident walking. Often, this is linked with a fear of falling. You do not trust your balance or your ability to respond quickly if you tripped, so you begin to avoid having to negotiate uneven surfaces, steps, slopes, mud. But this is an ever-closing circle and you can reach the point where you stop going out at all because you no longer enjoy walking.

Nordic walking can help you break this cycle and regain your balance and confidence. It feels easier than regular walking because the poles act as support, then all of a sudden you notice that you're standing taller, your balance is better, your joints don't hurt and you've started enjoying walking again.

Some good warm-up exercises to get you walking confidently are:

🌿 Open/close

🌿 Leg swings

🌿 Heel/toe roll

🌿 Ankle circles

Top Tips

- **Check your shoes.** This might seem a small point, but the weight of your entire body balances over your feet, so do all you can to make sure they – and you – are well supported by your footwear. Your shoes must fit properly, so they cannot be worn down and must be flexible enough for you to roll from your heel through your foot to your toes. If you wear shoes with laces, be sure to do them up properly so that your foot is not slipping about in your shoe, which could throw you off balance. Comfortable feet equal a comfortable walk.

- **Start small.** You do not have to walk for long. Just by being out you have overcome the biggest barrier: getting started. Start small and build up. One of the best ways to begin is to walk a short set route from your front door, this could just be to the end of the street and back. Build your confidence with Nordic walking poles, then start increasing your distance. Tracking your progress is a great motivator. See the section on goal setting in chapter eight for more information.

- **Walk on firm surfaces.** If you are just starting out, walking on tarmac or other firm surfaces is easier than walking over uneven ground. Once your confidence builds, stepping out over bumpy ground greatly strengthens your ankles and helps improve balance.

- **Head up, eyes down.** Dropping your head to look down and watch your feet just pulls you closer to the ground you are trying to avoid. There are of course some situations where you'll need to look at the ground, but this should be the exception, not the rule. Keep your head lifted and use your eyes to scan the ground ahead, anticipating what your feet will be treading over. This will improve your proprioception (your sense of your body, its movement and position) and help your balance. When you walk with your head up, you should just be able to see your foot peeking into view in your peripheral vision. If you can see your whole foot, you have dropped your head.

- **Breathe using the rhythm of your poles.** Counting your breath in and out in rhythm with your pole plant is a good way to develop a strong walking pattern and build confidence.

- **Lift your toes and 'squeeze lemons' under your feet.** Your heel/toe action will increase the blood supply to your ankles, feet and lower body muscles, strengthening them and improving flexibility. Imagine squeezing a lemon under your foot with each step.

- **A firm pole placement.** Placing your pole with confidence and pushing firmly down will give you greater stability and strengthen your abdominal muscles, which play a central role in good balance.

- **Relax your shoulders.** Roll your shoulders back and down. Wiggle your head to release any tension in your neck. Dissipating tension in your body can help reduce anxiety and improve your balance.

- **Build some balance exercises into your walk.** See below for two clever little exercises that take barely any time and will help improve your balance. With Nordic walking, you can use your poles to steady yourself while doing these if you need to.

- **Join a Nordic walking group.** There are many lovely Nordic walking instructors and welcoming and friendly groups. Regular contact with a good instructor will ensure your technique is good; plus, joining a group and creating a social event around your Nordic walking will benefit your mental health.

Common mistakes

- **Holding the poles upright** instead of angling them backward. This makes it harder to maintain good posture.

- **Breathing high in your chest** instead of down and lifting your shoulders as you breathe in creates tension in your neck. Shallow breathing can also increase anxiety.

- **Taking small nervous steps** and not using your feet properly.

- **Scrunching up your toes** in your shoes – this will destabilise you and inhibit a correct foot roll.

BALANCE EXERCISES

Once we pass fifty, we should be building daily balance exercises into our lives. Here are three ways you can improve your balance:

- **Stand on one leg.** Research has shown that your ability to stand on one leg is a powerful predictor of how long you will live. In one study, people over fifty who were unable to stand on one leg for ten seconds or longer were over 80% more likely to die within a decade.[55] Doing a single leg stand while cleaning your teeth will ensure you build it into your daily routine. If you find a single leg stand easy, do it with your eyes closed.

- **Walk a straight line**, placing the heel of one foot directly in front of the toes of the other foot. Walk at least twenty steps. Now do this in reverse, walking backward. If you find this easy, try doing it with your eyes closed.

- **Roll your bare feet over and around a tennis ball.** It's a wonderful massage for your feet and will improve your foot health and flexibility, which in turn will boost your balance.

TRISH'S STORY

I've always been prone to falling or tripping, due to problems with weak ankles, knees and a bad back. For years, I wasn't able to walk much further than two or three miles before seizing up. Then, one autumn, while working in the garden I fell and damaged the peroneal nerve in my left leg. This left me in a lot of pain and with drop foot on my left side. The orthopaedic surgeon explained that an operation would probably make things worse and referred me for physiotherapy. After six months, not much had changed and my physiotherapist suggested that I try Nordic walking. I'd never heard of it but, desperate to find something that would help, I gave it a go. I've never looked back.

I joined the local Nordic walking club where I basically learned how to walk properly again. Not only was my left foot improving but, as Nordic walking uses every muscle in your body, I was getting much fitter. So much so that, two years later, I took part in the Three Peaks Challenge in Wales and walked up Sugar Loaf Mountain – 596 metres high. I'll never forget the elation I felt when I reached the top. My friends and family were absolutely amazed – I could now join them on walks without seizing up and didn't trip or fall while out shopping.

I now Nordic walk regularly, in any weather. I have also met some wonderful people from all walks of life, of mixed ages and abilities, and have made some truly special friends. During the pandemic, Nordic walking was so important during those early months when we were only allowed out once a day. I could Nordic walk from my front door and exercise my whole body – it kept me fit and boosted my spirits. Once we were able to meet up outside again, I was able to join fellow Nordic walking friends for some much-needed socialising and exercise combined.

Nordic walking has totally transformed and enriched my life and I can't recommend it highly enough to anyone and everyone.

....

Menopause and strengthening your pelvic floor

The menopause can assault you from all directions – mood, weight, energy, joints, brain fog, body shape, sleep, bone health, pelvic floor – the list goes on. Figuring out how to manage it can be confusing, but studies have shown that regular exercise can significantly reduce menopausal symptoms and improve wellbeing.[56] Walking and breathing in time with your pole action is also relaxing and meditative, which can help alleviate the stress and anxiety often associated with menopause.

The holistic, balanced, supportive nature of Nordic walking makes it ideal if you are peri-menopausal or menopausal. First, it can help with weight loss and weight management. You can get your heart rate up and burn more calories than walking but without pounding your joints through jogging. Nordic walking is also a whole-body strengthening exercise, which is perfect for trimming inches and toning, especially those hard to tackle areas such as the upper arms and waist.

As a weight-bearing exercise, it is good for keeping your bones strong and healthy and I've been astonished at the number of clients who've said it's had a positive impact on their pelvic floor function. Your diaphragm, spine muscles, core abdominal muscles that wrap around your middle, and your pelvic floor all work together as one unit to protect, support and improve your body's overall movement. Like a trampoline, it is designed to be elastic and it can be tightened and released as needed.

Some great exercises to use if you're Nordic walking to manage menopause and strengthen your pelvic floor are:

- Shoulder rolls
- Pelvic rocks
- Rear toe taps

Top tips

- **For stress-reduction.** Walking and breathing in time with your pole action is relaxing and meditative.

- **For fitness and weight loss.** Nordic walk at least three times a week and include a long walk together with shorter faster walks. See chapter nine for more information.

- **For toning and strengthening.** Single-arm and double-arm polling, plus slowing your walking speed down are all ways you can increase your muscle tone and strength. Look back to chapter nine for specific tips.

- **Focus on your pelvic floor.** Spend five minutes of your walk focusing on your pelvic floor. Relax your pelvic floor sling as you breathe in and tighten it as you breathe out. It doesn't matter if you don't think anything is happening, just by taking your attention to that area you will be working it, even if you don't feel it. Piggy-backing some pelvic floor exercises onto your Nordic walking makes it easy to build them into your life.

- **Engage but don't brace your core.** Drawing your belly button in gently toward your spine as you walk is an effective way of engaging your core abdominal muscles and protecting your lower back. But over-tightening these muscles (bracing) can bear down on your pelvic floor and weaken it. It can also impact your breathing and movement pattern. If you tend to over-tighten your belly, try relaxing it as you breathe in and tightening it on each exhale.

- **Breathe with your diaphragm.** Your diaphragm is part of the deep core cylinder of muscles protecting and supporting your body. Using this muscle for breathing will strengthen and support the rest of the cylinder, including your pelvic floor. Look back to Step Two in chapter four for reminders on breathing.

- **Rotate.** Gently rotating your upper body will encourage your spine and pelvis to work together and help strengthen your pelvic floor.

- **Heel/toe roll.** An active heel/toe roll will help engage your glutes and the whole back (posterior) line of your body. This back line connects through your pelvis where your pelvic floor muscles are attached. Many of the pelvic floor muscles sit toward the back, so when you heel/toe roll actively you feed muscle energy through the whole back line of your body, energising your pelvic floor.

- **Stretch your adductors.** The muscles of your inner thigh play an important role in the health and effectiveness of your pelvic floor and need to be regularly stretched, as Minia Alonso explains below.

Common mistakes

Not prioritising yourself. Women typically look after other people's needs before their own, but menopause is a time when you must prioritise your health. Doing so will get your body into the best possible shape for the next chapter of your life and will enable you to give more effectively to others. Schedule your walks into your diary and make a commitment to walk with friends or attend a regular Nordic walking class.

The impact of the menopause can hit hard and affect all areas of your life. It can feel a lonely path sometimes. From my experience, I encourage you to just keep walking. Whether it is fast and furious or slow and mindful, walking soothes and strengthens, and works in harmony with your body.

EXPERT VIEW: MINIA ALONSO, REMEDIAL MASSAGE PRACTIONER

Pelvic floor

The pelvic floor is a sling of twelve muscles (in three layers) underneath your pelvis. It runs from your tailbone at the back to your pubic bone at the front and is connected on the sides by your sit bones, creating a trampoline-like base for your body. Both men and women have a pelvic floor, it's just talked about more with women because of the effect that pregnancy and childbirth has on it.

Stability in your pelvic floor is an integral part of your deep core strength, spine control and breathing and is key to avoiding problems with incontinence and prolapse. For stability, your pelvic floor needs to be strong but not rigid. It requires you to combine two apparently different things: resilience and movement. Successfully balancing these two components is the key to healthy function.

A healthy pelvic floor allows you to control your bowel movements and urination, and to enjoy sexual intercourse. For all of this, you need your pelvic floor to be dynamic, able to fully release or fully engage, and to switch readily back and forth between these two states as you breathe and walk. This dynamic balance must be established before you can work at strengthening your pelvic floor.

To get a sense of how this works, imagine yourself jumping on a trampoline. The webbed fabric acts as a shock absorber. It is strong and yet springy. One moment it stretches and the next it springs back. But what if the fabric of the trampoline was pulled down and held, preventing it from springing back? The trampoline no longer works. This can happen to our pelvic floor and, over time, can lead to weakness in its muscles. Exactly how does this happen?

Until recently, it was thought that a weak pelvic floor was one that literally allows things to fall through the pelvis. You may still come across this view, which is rooted in outdated anatomical thinking that lacked an appreciation of bio tensegrity. In the pre-bio tensegrity understanding, the body was seen as a stack of components – bones stacked one on top of one other with gravity pulling down. In this world, if anything fell it needed pushing back up via the tightening of muscles. The modern view is different.

Over the last forty years, the steady development of myofascial science has been moving us away from the idea of stacked components and toward the idea that our bodies rely on the balance of tension (bio tensegrity). Our bodies are actually built with a dynamic suspension system, a fascial web that encases everything (muscles, bones, organs) within it. Our body shape is maintained by a balance of tension across this entire structure. Within this system, things cannot fall, so what might seem like a weakness in the pelvic floor can in fact be too much tension in the nearby soft tissue, pulling our suspension system out of alignment. In this situation, as hard as we try to relax our pelvic floor, it may be impossible for us to do so effectively until we can find the source of tension within the pelvis.

Where does this tension come from? Often, through tightness in the abdomen, adductors, deep hip rotators, glutes and feet fascially pulling on the pelvic floor. There are lots of ways that tension can get into the system. It could be an injury, such as a fall or a knock to the pelvis, or a chronic movement disfunction such as an issue in the foot, ankle, or knee that causes you to limp. Over time, these things can build up tension within the pelvis. Emotional trauma and stress can also cause tension. That feeling you get in the pit of your stomach when you receive bad news, or you're about to go into a high-stress situation, this causes physical tension in the pelvic tissues. In women, any kind of scar tissue from labour can cause a three-dimensional pull through the pelvis and its surrounding areas. Poor posture can also introduce tension to your pelvis.

To bring your internal suspension system back into balance, it is important to look at all the structures that connect to the pelvis – the abdomen, adductors, deep hip rotators and glutes – and also the structures that work in synergy with the pelvic floor, such as your diaphragm. Keeping these muscles flexible, strong and healthy will give you a dynamic, elastic pelvic floor that can readily engage and release as needed.

Older adults

Not doing any physical activity is bad, no matter what your age or health status, but exercise becomes even more important as you age. By sheer dint of getting older we lose muscle mass (3–8% per decade after the age of thirty, and even more after the age of sixty)[57] and our bone health, balance, flexibility and co-ordination wane too.

Doing something about this can be daunting and sometimes it's hard to know where to begin. If your fitness has declined, there's the added anxiety of whether you can reverse the slump and rebuild it.

Most research says it's never too late to start exercising and that improvements in heart health, joint mobility, muscle strength, balance and flexibility are possible at any age. In one heart study, a group of sixty-one healthy but inactive adults aged forty-five to sixty-four were able to increase their heart elasticity by 25% simply through starting an exercise regime.[58] Not everything is possible. You can't, for instance, reverse an osteo-arthritic joint. But you can keep that joint moving, build up your strength in the supporting muscles, and ensure that your circulation is delivering as many nutrients to that area as possible.

As I've already discussed, Nordic walking is an ideal exercise as you get older. It's outdoors, sociable, easy to learn, supportive, good for your posture, kind on your joints, improves your balance and works your whole body. You are never too old to start Nordic walking. If you can walk, you can Nordic walk.

Some of the things that Nordic walking can help you achieve, which are often a struggle for those in their later years, include:

- Walking with friends and family and going upstairs without feeling puffed out.
- Being able to put your coat on and reach for your car seatbelt strap easily.
- For women, being able to do your bra strap up at the back.
- Standing on one leg to put your socks on.
- Reaching down to tie your shoelaces and cut your toenails.
- Carrying bags comfortably.
- Having the stamina to play with your grandchildren all day long.

The best exercises to warm up with to get the most out of Nordic walking as you age are:

- Chin slides
- Open/close
- Kayaking
- Leg swings
- Heel/toe roll

Top tips

- **Do warm-up exercises.** Feeling a bit stiff and sore is a typical feature of getting older. Leg swings and big arm movements like the open/close and kayaking recommended above will get your joints moving, your blood circulating and set you up for a beneficial walk.

- **Keep your shoulders wide.** Rolling your shoulders back and down and lifting your ribs up will stop you stooping, make breathing easier and free up your arm swing. Re-read chapter three for more tips on posture.

- **Keep your head lifted.** Slide your head back as far as feels comfortable (the chin slide warm-up exercise can be done while you're walking) and lift it up and away from your shoulders. Your body will be better aligned, which will make walking more comfortable.

- **Keep your feet active.** Lifting your toe and using your foot rockers to propel you forward will improve your foot health and flexibility and your foot and leg circulation. Squeeze those lemons under your feet as you walk.

- **Keep your arms and hands active.** Swinging your arms will help with your speed and upper body rotation (and general back health). At the same time, gently squeezing and relaxing your hand round the grip will improve your circulation. If you have arthritic hands, integrated glove straps will spread the load over your hand.

- **Aim for two-and-a-half hours of exercise per week.** The UK Chief Medical Officers say that doing two-and-a-half hours of moderate-intensity exercise can make a big difference to your physical and mental health.[59] Physical activity also plays a key role in keeping your brain healthy.

- **Join a group.** Nordic walking with others is fun and sociable and helps you meet the recommended weekly exercise targets.

- **Stretch.** Stretching at the end of your walk will help maintain and even increase your flexibility and joint mobility so that you can walk regularly and keep active.

- **Know your limits.** While Nordic walking is a safe exercise, it is wise not to try and do too much too soon. Keep checking in with yourself on how you're feeling and stop for a rest if you need to. If you are on medication, especially heart medication, wearing a heart rate monitor won't necessarily give you an accurate reading of how hard you're working, so use the Talk Test in chapter eight and pay attention to your body's physical cues. If you haven't exercised in a long while, have had a fall, or are on lots of medication, talk to your doctor before you start Nordic walking.

Common mistakes

- **Not pushing through your strap** as you won't be strengthening your arms and upper body.

- **Taking small steps.** Be confident with your heel/toe roll and your stride length will automatically increase.

Improving how you walk will improve how you feel – it's never too late to start.

ELEVEN

Looking After Your Body

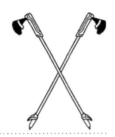

This group of menus focuses on some of the key functions that help keep us fit and well: a healthy back and joints, heart and circulation, and strong bones.

Love your joints

It's easy to let sore joints narrow your fitness parameters or lower your expectations of what you are capable of. Walking, especially Nordic walking, is an excellent way to keep your joints moving and the supporting muscles strong. The feel-good endorphins released when you get your heart rate up and exercise outside can also reduce any discomfort you feel. The social nature of Nordic walking makes it fun, too.

What I've noticed about Nordic walking for people with sore joints in particular is that, as well as establishing good posture, the technique encourages a symmetrical, even walking pattern. You'd be surprised how many people unconsciously shift their weight over to one side to protect a sore knee or hip. Unfortunately, while it might ease the immediate hip/knee pain, it throws your body out of balance, which can trigger all sorts of other problems and joint strains. When your body is properly aligned, your weight passes down through your body evenly and your joints can move naturally without stress. This all amounts to an integrated and smooth walking experience that keeps your joints mobile, strengthens the supporting muscles and returns the joy of walking.

If you have arthritis and have been inactive for a while, or have any anxiety about exercising, speak to a health professional before you start Nordic walking. Some great exercises that can help ease you in and get you started are:

- Sky reaches
- Shoulder rolls
- Open/close
- Leg swings
- Heel/toe roll
- Ankle circles

Top tips

- **Think about the walking surface.** Choose a surface that's kind on your joints. Tarmac and hard surfaces are unforgiving. Walking on stony, slippy and uneven ground is also tough on your joints as these surfaces can jolt or stress them. The kindest surfaces for those with joint concerns are well-conditioned short grass or dirt tracks.

- **Start slowly.** It takes a while for stiff joints to warm up, especially when it's cold, so start slowly and gradually increase your movement as your joints become more mobile. Stopping to do additional mobilisation exercises is also helpful.

- **Walk with good alignment and maintain an even weight distribution.** Lengthen your spine, lift your chest and maintain a good head position so that your weight flows smoothly through your back and joints. Keep the pressure through your poles and the weight over your feet even between your left and right sides.

- **Use an integrated glove strap.** If you have arthritis in your hands, you may find wearing a glove that has the strap integrated within it more comfortable. See chapter seven for more detail. You can also keep just a light grip on the poles and rely entirely on the strap.

- **Keep your upper body moving.** Swinging your arms, softly squeezing and relaxing your hands around the pole grip and building in a gentle natural rotation will improve your circulation and the synovial fluid to your joints.

- **Heel first.** The heel/toe roll, especially the lifting of your toes as you step forward, will help mobilise your ankle and encourage the blood supply to that area. If you have arthritis in your feet, speak to a health professional before taking up Nordic walking.

- **Think middle toe for sore knees.** If you have turned-out feet and sore knees, you may find it helps to 'think middle toe' as you roll through your foot and push off with your toes. Many of my clients have said this has helped with their knee pain.

- **Be careful going downhill.** Ensuring the correct technique when going downhill will lessen the pressure through your knees. Keep the poles angled backward, soften your knees, engage your core, and keep your weight between your heel and mid-foot. See the section on walking downhill in chapter eight for further tips.

- **Increase your distance slowly.** Don't be tempted to push yourself too hard and risk aggravating symptoms.

Common mistakes

- ◊ **Walking with upright poles.** Nordic walking requires you to angle the poles backward. You won't get the full benefits for your joints if you walk with them upright.

- ◊ **Over-reaching with your leading foot.** Keep a normal stride pattern to avoid unnecessary pressure on your joints.

- ◊ **Planting the pole in the ground too firmly.** This could jar your wrists and shoulders.

- ◊ **Flexing your wrist as you push through the strap.** Keep your wrist firm so that the power flows through your wrists and doesn't aggravate them.

Our bodies were designed to move. Exercise and arthritis can and should coexist. People with arthritis who exercise regularly have less pain, more energy, improved sleep and better day-to-day function.

Your joints may feel uncomfortable or sore after exercising, especially if you have been inactive for some time. This is normal and does not mean that you are harming your joints, but if you are worried, see a health professional.

Better back

Nordic walking is the exercise of choice for many people with bad backs. Clients have told me that just having the poles in their hands lifts their body up and makes them better aligned. Walking in the Nordic way, using their arms, shoulders and upper back and engaging their core and lower body more effectively, has helped them reduce stress in and on their body and ease neck and back pain. With the correct technique, they have been able to walk fast and long distances, all the while being supported and propelled forward by the poles.

This is not surprising. Research and medics consider walking to be one of the best forms of exercise for back health (see chapter three for the science) and Nordic walking is just an enhanced form of regular walking: holistic, symmetrical and supportive, raising your heart rate, and pumping feel-good hormones round your body.

These exercises are fantastic for your back; do them if you can:

- Shoulder rolls
- Open/close
- Kayaking
- Sky reaches
- Pelvic rocks
- Leg swings
- Rear toe taps

Top Tips

- **Avoid hard walking surfaces** where possible, or those which might jar your back, like stony or slippery ground.

- **Walk tall using the power of four**: stand tall, chin level, shoulders down and chest lifted. This will put you in the correct postural position and strengthen those crucial postural muscles.

- **Pull your belly button slightly toward your spine**; this can ease back tension and help maintain good walking posture.

- **Walk lightly.** Your spine and lower back are affected by the impact of your feet on the ground. Lifting your toe, dropping your heel gently to the ground, and actively rolling through your foot to push off with your toes will produce a smooth foot action that is kind on your back.

- **Push back with your thigh to fire your glutes.** If you don't use your glutes to propel you forward, your lower back muscles often take over the job, causing strain and pain. Pushing your thigh back as you toe-off with your back foot is a neat way to engage your glutes, stretch your hip flexors and protect your back.

- **Push through the pole.** Every time you place the pole in the ground you switch on your core. The longer you keep that downward force, the harder your core works and the more it strengthens, protecting and supporting your lower back.

- **Rotate.** The gentle natural rotation as you walk boosts circulation the whole way down your spine and sends more oxygen and nutrients to the discs and vertebrae.

- **Belly breathe.** Breathing from your upper chest generally results in your shoulders lifting and increased neck and shoulder tension. Breath down into your belly instead. You can also use your breath to relax and de-stress – see the section on mindfulness in chapter ten for more on this.

- **Keep a steady pace.** Nordic walking is a gentle body movement. There's nothing 'fast and furious' to upset your back. Keep a steady pace going so that your back warms into the rhythm and then try and walk for at least forty minutes, especially if it's a cold day, to reap the full benefits from the Nordic walking movement.

Get out of breath. We store a great deal of our emotions and worries in our backs. Raising your heart rate and getting out of breath releases endorphins, serotonin, dopamine and other chemicals that help reduce stress, boost mood and relieve pain.

Common mistakes

Dropping your head. This piles stress onto your neck and shoulders. Stand tall, with your chin level and slide your ears back toward your shoulders.

Slouching. This weakens your mid-back muscles and contributes to back ache. Keep your chest proud and your shoulders wide.

Raising your shoulders as you push through the pole.

Swinging your hips from side to side. This puts strain on your lower back – keep your hips level.

Walking with too much or too little curve in your lower back. Do the pelvic rocks warm-up to find what's called a 'neutral' spine.

Nordic walking in and of itself may be enough to alleviate back pain, but most of my clients have found that it's best done in conjunction with some other form of back care, so consider seeing a chiropractor, osteopath or physiotherapist.

Circulation and heart health

If you want a healthy heart and good circulation, a total body exercise like Nordic walking is ideal. It gets your heart rate up, the blood pumping around your body and the energy flowing from the tips of your fingers to the tops of your toes. I no longer get numb fingers since Nordic walking regularly and, bucking the family trend, not a single varicose vein has returned since my last operation over six years ago.

Being active provides a good supply of nutrients and oxygen for your brain, muscles and cells. Your heart gets physically stronger and your blood pressure and cholesterol can drop.

The best news is that you can get the benefit of all of this without having to go crazy with effort or get hot and sweaty in a gym. With Nordic walking alone, all of these benefits can be yours; this is something you can do while chatting to friends and enjoying the great outdoors.

If you have a diagnosed heart condition check with your doctor that it's safe to take up Nordic walking and if there are any exercise restrictions. For instance, adding inclines such as hills may raise your heart rate too high and could be dangerous. You also need to keep track of your exercise intensity. Heart rate monitors may not give an accurate reading of how hard you are working as heart medication can artificially reduce your heart rate, so speak to an expert about what heart rate range you should be aiming for and use the Talk Test to self-monitor (see chapter eight). If you're walking with friends, this makes doing the Talk Test easy. Remember to never ignore pain, especially chest pain.

To boost circulation and improve heart health, incorporate these warm-up exercises into your Nordic walking routine:

- Sky reaches
- Open/close
- Kayaking

Top tips

- **Squeeze your hand round the pole handle** as you swing your arm forward; this acts as a pump, returning the blood back up your veins to your heart. You'll have toasty fingers in the winter and no fat fingers in hot weather.

- **Work your feet.** Dynamically rolling from your heel through to your toes helps push the blood back up your legs to your heart.

- **Build a breathing rhythm.** Your lungs are crucial to good circulation. Long and deep is better than short and shallow. Use the rhythm of your poles to build a good breathing rhythm.

- **Keep a steady pace.** You don't have to walk fast to improve your heart health. A comfortable, steady pace will allow your heart chambers to completely fill and your heart to become more efficient.

- **Include hills and intervals to raise your heart rate fast.** Adding inclines, intervals and pace walks are quick ways to up your heart rate, strengthen your heart wall and get your circulation going.

Common mistakes

- **Forgetting about posture.** Good posture promotes good circulation. Stand tall, chest proud, shoulders back. Your chest houses your heart and lungs. Good posture gives them room to work properly.

- **Forgetting about technique.** Lifting you toes and squeezing your hands round the pole grip act as venous return pumps, boosting your circulation. Swinging your arms and bringing in a natural rotation is a great way to get your upper body moving and the blood pumping round your body.

- **Doing too much too fast.** Build up gradually and monitor intensity. It's always sensible to build up your walk time and intensity gradually to avoid putting undue strain on your body, but this is especially important if you have a heart condition.

Regular walking can help increase heart elasticity, reduce cardiac stiffness (a cause of heart failure) and lessen almost all of the most common risk factors for heart disease.[60] It's never too late to start.

Supporting strong bones

As a weight-bearing, muscle-strengthening exercise, Nordic walking helps build and maintain strong bones. It also improves co-ordination, joint mobility, posture and balance and so makes you more steady on your feet (four legs are better than two), helping to prevent falls and consequent fractures.

Bone is living tissue and becomes stronger with exercise. If you have been diagnosed with osteoporosis or have risk factors, the Royal Osteoporosis Society says you should do more exercise, not less.[61] Nordic walking is an outdoor, holistic exercise based entirely on your regular walking. Its whole-body nature improves circulation and makes it an excellent weight-bearing activity if you are worried about your bone health and osteoporosis and, because the poles act as a support, you will be able to walk further with seemingly less effort.

Nordic walking is especially suitable for those with osteoporosis because it uses both the upper and lower body in the act of walking, pulling on the majority of the muscles in your body to help propel you forward. The technique integrates with your natural walking movement and strengthens your postural muscles, helping to keep your skeleton aligned and strong.

If you have osteoporosis or fragile bones, check with your doctor or health professional that Nordic walking is suitable for you, and then make sure you do appropriate warm-up exercises. The ones I recommend are:

- Chin slides
- Shoulder rolls
- Leg swings

Top tips

- **Power through your strap.** The correct Nordic walking technique involves pushing through the strap to propel you forward. This strengthens your wrists, arms and mid-back area. The downward pressure you apply through your poles strengthens the deep abdominal muscles, supporting your spine.

- **Keep your weight even.** Make sure that you're not leaning your weight over to one side as this will put your skeleton out of alignment.

- **Use your breathing to release tension.** Muscle tension inhibits the smooth working of your body and makes it difficult to walk with good posture. Establish a steady breathing rhythm and use it to drain away tension.

- **Seek out hills.** Walking uphill is more demanding on your muscles, increasing their pull on your bones and helping to strengthen them.

- **Add exercises.** Adding walking lunges, squats and a few press-ups against a tree or park bench can all boost your muscle and bone strength.

- **Expose your skin to sunlight.** This triggers your body to make vitamin D which is essential for healthy bones. In the UK the sun is only strong enough during the summer months for this to happen, so make the most of it and roll up your sleeves (don't forget your sun-cream though).

- **Carry a water bottle or light weight on your back.** In a talk on spine health given by a nurse from a fractures clinic, she recommended carrying a small water bottle at shoulder blade height to boost spine health.

Common mistakes

- **Slouching and/or dropping your head.** Not standing tall with your chest proud compresses your vertebrae, and dropping your head pulls your whole spine out of alignment. This is bad for your muscles and bones. Stand tall, shoulders back and down, head in neutral, chest proud, hips level.

- **Nordic walking with vertical poles.** You won't get the upper body benefits.

- **Bending over at the waist when walking uphill.** This puts immense stress on your lower back.

Strengthening your bones is important at every stage of life but it takes on extra urgency as you get older and after the menopause. By simply Nordic walking regularly, you can improve your bone health and reduce your risk of fractures.

TWELVE

Health Conditions

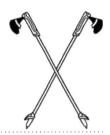

Being diagnosed with a health condition is a time when many people look to start exercising more. The group of menus provided in this chapter contain tips on how Nordic walking can support you through a cancer journey, with Parkinson's, asthma or COPD (chronic obstructive pulmonary disease), or if you have diabetes. Nordic walking is holistic wellbeing activity that can help improve your mental and physical health and support you throughout all of life's trials and tribulations.

Keeping active through cancer

Keeping active during and after treatment for cancer can help manage some of the side effects of treatment, improve your energy levels, boost your physical recovery and support your mental wellbeing. Getting and staying active can also help protect against future cancers, especially bowel and breast cancer.[62]

Studies have shown that Nordic walking is a safe and effective exercise for people with cancer and I have trained many people during and after their cancer treatment, as well as developing a Nordic walking with cancer programme for the national cancer charity Penny Brohn UK.

If your balance has been affected by treatment or your joints are sore, Nordic walking provides multiple benefits. The poles help steady you, and pushing them backward using the straps strengthens your deep core stabilising muscles, which assist with balance. Using poles also reduces pressure on sore joints by spreading the load. This is particularly beneficial when walking downhill.

If you have had breast cancer you may have had the lymph nodes under your armpit partially or entirely removed during surgery, resulting in lymphedema. The pendulum swing and hand squeeze round the pole handle in the Nordic walking technique, when coupled with good breathing, helps drain the lymph. I have had frequent comments from clients about how Nordic walking has improved their lymphedema and peripheral neuropathy. The arm swing action also increases the blood flow to the whole shoulder and chest area, assisting healing.

Some great warm-up exercises to incorporate into your Nordic walking practice when undergoing or following treatment for cancer are:

- Shoulder rolls
- Open/close
- Rear toe taps
- Ankle circles

Top tips

- **Seek help.** Before you begin, speak to one of the cancer health professionals supporting you and discuss your plans with them. Although physical activity is recommended for people with cancer, there are many different types of cancer and each person's treatment journey will vary.

- **Work around your medication.** Go out when you know your energy level will be higher.

- **Chest up, shoulders back.** Following the posture tips in chapter three, especially lifting your chest and rolling your shoulders back and down, will help move you away from a closed, rounded (protective) posture, which you may have unconsciously adopted following your cancer diagnosis and/or treatment. Just this postural shift alone can feel empowering.

- **Breathe down and away** from your shoulders and out sideways. This will help you de-stress, release tension in your neck and shoulder area and support your lymphatic system.

- **Adopt a rhythmic natural arm swing.** If you have breast cancer, the Nordic walking arm swing is an excellent way of boosting the circulation around your chest and shoulder area and encourage lymph drainage. Don't overdo it, though, a comfortable pendulum arm swing from your shoulder is sufficient.

- **Walk your hands up and down** the shaft of one of your poles as an additional warm-up exercise.

- **Minimise vibration up the pole shaft.** If you have had breast cancer or surgery around your shoulder area, try to minimise vibration up the pole shaft as this has the potential to jar up your arm. You can do this by using 100% carbon poles if possible and walking on soft even surfaces like grass.

- **Push through the strap.** Pushing through your Nordic walking strap during your backward arm swing will engage and strengthen your core stability and maximise balance benefits. You will also involve your upper body muscles more fully, supporting bone strength. Again, don't overdo it. Only use as much power as feels comfortable.

Walk mindfully. Anxiety and depression are common side effects of cancer. The endorphins released just by getting outside and being active can spark a shift to a more positive mood, as can walking mindfully. Harmonising your steps with your breathing is rhythmic and soothing for your body. Concentrating on your Nordic walking technique gives your brain something to focus on, helping keep other worries at bay.

Keep an exercise diary. Keep a record of how active you've been and how you feel so you can see your progress.

Common mistakes

Expecting too much too soon. Going for a daily walk, even if just ten minutes, will have big health benefits. I know from clients that even this can be challenging sometimes, so be kind on yourself. Start small and work from there, knowing that you will have high and low energy days and that even on a good day, your energy levels can drop quickly. Macmillan advises that if possible you should gradually build up to the recommended physical activity guidelines. You might find their resource booklet 'Physical activity and cancer' a useful source of information and inspiration.[63]

Not swinging your arms properly. Ensure you're swinging your arm freely from your shoulder and that it's not clamped to your side, for maximum lymphatic drainage benefits. Don't worry if the poles bounce or drag over the ground, this will improve with time and practice.

An often overlooked aspect of cancer is its impact on carers. This is an emotionally demanding role and it is sometimes hard to find things that you can still do together.

Nordic walking is suitable for all fitness levels and can be done in any location, urban or rural. Learning something new together is not only a good distraction from a challenging time but is fun and rewarding in its own right.

PAT'S STORY

I was diagnosed with breast cancer and had a lumpectomy followed by chemotherapy, radiotherapy and hormone tablets. I tried to keep positive throughout, but I felt wrecked much of the time. Sometimes it was an effort just to walk to the bathroom. Moving my arm was difficult because I'd had lymph nodes removed, and I was in constant pain from nerve damage to my arm.

I heard about Vicky's Nordic walking with cancer group from my haematology and oncology centre and I attended my first session while still undergoing treatment. I didn't know what to expect, but I wanted to build some type of physical activity into my life and I liked the sound of Nordic walking.

Vicky explained how Nordic walking works and what I could expect from the walk, sorting out the right poles for me and putting me at my ease. Another beginner was there and Vicky took both of us to a quiet area of the park and taught us the basic Nordic walking technique. Although it's based on your normal walking pattern, I had to concentrate on how I was walking and the time went by in a flash. Being outside and focusing on something other than my cancer was a wonderful distraction.

Nordic walking helped me on the road to getting fit, feeling healthy, getting outdoors and taking time to look at nature and appreciate the small things in life, like simply feeling the wind on my face. It has not only been good for my health and wellbeing, but it has lifted my spirits. I enjoyed the social side, meeting other people dealing with cancer, sharing our concerns and cancer journeys and how we were coping with the side effects of treatment. I always looked forward to the group class and, now that I've returned to work, I still meet up and Nordic walk with the friends that I made.

Walking well with Parkinson's

Parkinson's UK say that exercise can be as important as your medication to help you take control and manage your symptoms.[64] In the first part of this book, I explained the science behind why Nordic walking is considered such a suitable exercise, but, briefly, the technique helps you to not slouch, supports you as you walk, propels you forward and ensures you maintain a good stride. As a skills-based exercise, learning how to Nordic walk and applying the technique will keep your brain active and challenged and your brain/body connection strong. It will help you keep up with friends and family and the skills you learn can be transferred to your regular walking, improving your confidence and posture.

One of my first Nordic walking clients was a keen walker who had Parkinson's. She was becoming increasingly frustrated that her balance was going, the range of her arm and leg movements was decreasing and that she was tiring quickly, even on a straightforward walk. It curtailed her enjoyment of walking and spoilt a much-loved shared pastime with her husband.

Through Nordic walking, she became more aware of her alignment, her heel/toe foot roll and her breathing. She used her poles to help build a steady walking rhythm and improve her arm swing, which in turn increased her stride length. The poles helped accelerate her forward, increase her confidence and improve her balance. She and her husband were able to enjoy walking together once again. I was deeply affected by her story and still think about her now, even though this was over twelve years ago. Nordic walking gave her back her mobility and her happiness in walking.

For those wanting to Nordic walk with Parkinson's, some excellent warm-up exercises to incorporate are:

- Shoulder rolls
- Open/close
- Pelvic rocks
- Leg swings
- Rear toe taps
- Heel/toe roll

Top tips

- **Walk around your medication.** Walk at a time of day when you know you have more energy and be aware of your own limitations. Speak to a health professional if you're unsure about starting Nordic walking.

- **Stand tall.** Use all the posture tips in the Nordic walking foundations part of the book to help you stand tall. It is especially important to lift your chest and roll your shoulders back and down. If your lower back region is stiff, the pelvic rock exercises and levelling your hips will help.

- **Use your mind to get going.** If you're having trouble getting started, visualise kicking an object to help with your leg movement and marching to help with your arm swing.

- **Make sure your weight is even** over both feet and that your feet aren't too close together. Pulling your tummy button in toward your spine and pushing down through the poles will give you greater stability and improve your balance.

- **Pushing the poles firmly back** will encourage a strong recoil forward and improve the range of your arm swing. Visualise your arms swinging like the pendulum of a clock.

- **Think large.** Stride length can often shorten with Parkinson's, so reach out with your leading foot farther than you think you need to. Lifting your toe toward your knee as you step forward and pushing off with your toes at the end of your stride will increase your walking momentum and stride length.

- **Relax your neck and shoulders** as much as possible to avoid adding tension to your movement. Keep your neck long and wiggle your head occasionally to release neck tension. Roll your shoulders back and down periodically as you walk. This stops your shoulders from rounding forward and helps stretch your chest and improve your breathing.

- **Focus on the rhythm of your poles** to ensure it is even, then use that and your breathing to keep your walking rhythm smooth and controlled.

- **Rotate your upper body** to keep your posture good and avoid the tendency to side lean. It also helps release tension in your upper back. If you find it difficult to include this movement in your walking, build some stops into your walk to do torso twists.

🌿 **Join a walking group.** Nordic walking in a group is supportive, fun and will make the time fly. Learning from a qualified instructor will help you get the most benefit from Nordic walking.

Common mistakes

🌿 **Trying to do it all at once.** The brain and body can only cope with so much at a time, so expect learning Nordic walking to be a gradual process. Start with co-ordinating your arms and legs, then work towards increasing your arm swing, establishing a breathing and walking rhythm, being active with your feet and pushing through the pole with greater power.

🌿 **Walking with flat feet.** Keep your foot roll active by visualising squeezing lemons under your feet.

🌿 **Having one lazy side.** You will almost certainly have one side that works better than the other. Use your 'good side' to help improve the arm action, leg swing and foot roll on your 'lazy side'.

🌿 **Small movements.** Make a conscious effort to keep your stride and arm swing long.

🌿 **Leaning backward.** Keep your momentum going forward.

Parkinson's UK says this about the benefits of physical activity: 'Being active for 2.5 hours a week can help manage Parkinson's symptoms, and has a positive impact both physically and mentally. Break sweat. Lift your mood. Live well with Parkinson's.'[65] Getting outside and Nordic walking, ideally with companions, is the perfect way to live well with Parkinson's.

Asthma and respiratory conditions

Nordic walking is especially good for people with asthma and if you're one of the UK's eight million asthma sufferers I'd urge you to give it a go.[66] First, it changes your posture, both by reminding you how you should be holding yourself when walking and by strengthening those key postural muscles as you Nordic walk. Good posture gives your lungs more space to do their job and puts your head, neck and shoulders in the best possible position to facilitate easy breathing. Being well aligned places less stress on your body in general, allowing your respiratory system to function more efficiently. Nordic walking regularly will facilitate a postural habit that can spill over into your daily life so that you're walking well all the time, without having to think about it. This, coupled with the poles acting as support, can give you the confidence to start exercising again.

Second, being physically active strengthens your lungs. Nordic walking may feel easy but it's actually quite demanding on the body because all your muscles – both upper and lower body – are being used to propel you forward. Your lungs have to work hard to supply the additional oxygen your muscles demand.

Finally, it's fun. We've all started fitness classes or signed up to the gym with good intentions, but why do we stop? Nordic walking is just so enjoyable. Ask most Nordic walkers and they'll say that an hour's walk is the quickest hour in their day. When something's fun, our bodies respond to it. Everything feels easier, more relaxed, more responsive. As someone once said, laughter is medicine – well, it certainly is for the lungs.

If you have asthma or another respiratory condition and want to use Nordic walking to keep your lungs healthy, I recommend the following warm-up exercises:

- Chin slides
- Shoulder rolls
- Open/close
- Pelvic rocks

Top tips

- **Always take your reliever medication** with you on a walk. You never know when you might need it. Watch for asthma symptoms and stop and take your reliever medication if symptoms appear.

- **Lift your head.** Your head position influences how you breathe. Slide your chin back and lift your head up and away from your shoulders.

- **Relax your jaw and neck.** Holding tension in your jaw, neck or shoulders will impact your breathing. Relax your jaw (don't worry, you'll still be able to talk and laugh), and wiggle your neck occasionally to release any build up of tension.

- **Having the right height Nordic walking poles** and angling them back correctly will keep your posture good and support your breathing.

- **Establish a breathing rhythm.** Use the beat of your poles striking the ground to establish a steady breathing rhythm. This will give you something to focus on and help reduce any breathing-related anxiety.

- **Build your fitness gradually.** You don't have to walk fast or take on big hills to increase your fitness through Nordic walking. Simply by using your upper body to push through the poles you will be raising your heart rate and building your lung strength, capacity and efficiency. When you're ready to go a bit faster or up slopes, you'll find that the poles provide excellent support and make it feel easy.

- **Don't be afraid of exercising.** Exercise releases mood-boosting endorphins and exercising outdoors in nature and the fresh air benefits our mental health. An outdoor environment is perfect if you are anxious about catching a virus like flu or Covid-19 that might affect your lungs.

Common mistakes

- **Forgetting to maintain good posture.** Keep checking in with your head, chest, and shoulder alignment. The most important gap in your body is the one between your hips and chest. This is especially true for those with respiratory conditions. Lift your chest up out of your hips and never let that gap close. You will immediately be able to breathe more easily.

- **Breathing through your mouth.** Breathe in through your nose if you can, especially when the weather's cold. Breathing through your mouth pulls cold, dry air into your lungs, which may irritate your airways.

GEOF'S STORY

I've had asthma for over twenty years. It's quite mild and I manage it pretty well – using my preventer inhaler twice a day, going to regular reviews with my asthma nurse and always keeping my reliever inhaler with me when I go out. It's only when I catch a cold or get the flu that my asthma gets worse, and I struggle to keep my symptoms under control.

Although generally I cope well with my asthma, it's made me a couch potato over the years. In the past, if I did too much exercise, like heavy housework or gardening, I'd get out of breath quickly and be gasping for air, so I avoided anything too strenuous.

My wife and I heard about a local Nordic walking group and were intrigued by the idea of a fitness activity that wasn't too strenuous, provided a whole-body workout in fresh air and was something we could do together.

The first class was lots of fun and we decided to continue Nordic walking regularly. It has done wonders for my asthma. I'm pleased to say I've only had to use my reliever inhaler once on a walk, which was while we were climbing quite a steep slope. Since then, I've done some pretty challenging slopes, but I've stopped wheezing and no longer need to rest before I reach the top. Better still, now that my posture is better, my breathing has improved greatly.

Although Covid created additional anxiety for someone like me with asthma, knowing I could Nordic walk outdoors and exercise my lungs was a big relief. Sometimes you can feel helpless to know what to do for the best, but with Nordic walking I feel like I've been able to take my lung health, fitness and mental wellbeing into my own hands.

Diabetes

Whichever way you look at it, if you have diabetes being physically active makes a huge positive difference to your health. It can help you reduce your weight, body mass index (BMI) and blood sugar levels. It can also increase the level of 'good' cholesterol (HDL) in your blood, which helps protect your arteries and heart.[67] If you have type two diabetes, exercising can help your body use insulin better by increasing insulin sensitivity.

There's so much choice when it comes to exercise that it can be hard to know what's best, but studies have shown that Nordic walking is a great option if you have diabetes. The poles support your weight and make walking more comfortable – particularly benefi-cial if your foot health has been affected – and, because you are using your whole body, Nordic walking burns more calories than regular walking. It's something you can do all year round, whatever the weather, and because you can chat to friends while exercising, the time goes by in a flash. If you've previously been more sedentary, all this makes it much easier to make a change. If you're diabetic and looking to build Nordic walking into your lifestyle, I recommend the following warm-up exercises:

- Sky reaches
- Kayaking
- Leg swings
- Ankle circles
- Heel/toe roll

Top tips

- **Check your feet and footwear.** Diabetes can impact on your foot health so you'll want to pay especially close attention to your footwear. Check your toenails are cut short, your socks don't rub and are made from wicking fabric to keep your feet dry and cool, and that your shoes fit well.

- **Create a habit.** Regular exercise is key to successful weight loss, muscle tone, feel-good endorphins and reduced blood sugar levels. Try to find a local Nordic walking group with a skilled instructor to help you get the most from Nordic walking, arrange to meet and walk with friends for additional walks, and prioritise both by carving out time in your diary. Your mental and physical health will benefit, you will have more energy and through weight loss it's even possible to put your diabetes into remission.[68]

- **Maintain good posture to protect your feet.** Good alignment while Nordic walking will stack your weight correctly over your joints and feet, putting them under the least amount of stress. Follow the top tips in chapter three on posture.

- **Use your feet correctly** while walking, with an active heel/toe roll, to mobilise all the joints in your feet, distribute your weight evenly and promote foot health. Remember to 'squeeze lemons' under your feet as you walk to get your joints working and the blood flowing.

- **Walk on an even surface** to make it easier on your feet. Well-maintained grassy parks and paved surfaces are best if you are worried about your feet. If you do walk on stony or slippery ground, take extra care.

- **Keep an eye on your blood sugar.** This will be affected by how long you walk for and how fast your pace is. Make sure you check your blood sugar levels before, during and after your walk, and take medication and a fast-acting carbohydrate with you in case you need it.

- **Push through your poles to lose weight.** You don't have to Nordic walk fast to tone up and lose weight. Just pushing through the poles and engaging your upper body in the act of walking will increase your energy expenditure and help trim and tone your arms and waist, common problem areas for those with diabetes.

- **Wear your medical ID.**

Common mistakes

- **Wearing shoes that are too stiff.** You need shoes with flexible soles to move your feet properly and get oxygen and energy to your foot joints.

- **Leaning to one side.** Try to keep your weight even over both feet; use the poles to help.

- **Thinking you must walk lots to make a difference.** Even a few minutes a day can make a big difference when it comes to decreasing insulin resistance and lowering glucose levels.

From my experience, most diabetic people who try Nordic walking are surprised by how simple and effective it is and most of all, how much fun they have. Giving it a go could transform your health and your life.

SUMMARY OF PART FOUR

The different Nordic walking menus I've provided in this part of the book mean you will be able to adapt your Nordic walking to your fitness, health and wellbeing needs on any particular day, week or month. You can switch between them, or even blend the menus together. I often use Nordic walking in different ways within one walk – walking fast to blast off pent-up energy, slowing down to focus on strength and tone, then finishing mindfully to re-connect with the world around me.

Within each menu, I have given you the most suitable warm-up exercises, some top tips relevant to your specific motivation for and use of Nordic walking, and highlighted some common mistakes to try and avoid. There is some inevitable overlap between some of these tips, as the nature of Nordic walking means it has multifaceted benefits for a plethora of people and purposes. My hope is that these menus will continue to serve you now and long into your Nordic walking future.

Conclusion

Our bodies must move to be healthy. In this book, I have shown you that Nordic walking is natural and dynamic, and can adapt to your needs and be your exercise for life.

The whole-body action and specialist poles with integrated glove-type strap are Nordic walking's distinguishing characteristics. I have explained how these features set it apart from trekking, make it both more supportive and dynamic than regular walking, and offer a low-impact alternative to running. I have also set out the research behind the health and fitness benefits of Nordic walking including for weight loss, heart health and pain relief.

You now have the four simple steps to getting started with Nordic walking: posture, breathing, walking action and active use of the poles. The first three steps are all directly transferable to your regular walking and the more you Nordic walk, the better your posture, breathing and regular walking will become. You also have four golden rules for using Nordic walking poles correctly. The first is using the right height poles to maintain a natural arm swing and activate the key upper body muscles without placing unwanted stress on your neck and shoulders. The second is to angle your poles backward, which again helps keep your arm swing natural and powers you forward with good posture. The third golden rule is to swing from your shoulder and the fourth is to push through the strap. These two rules add power to your Nordic walking and trigger the engagement of your upper body in the act of walking.

I have explained the different types of Nordic walking poles and discussed the ideal clothing and footwear, so that you can be confident you are properly prepared for Nordic walking. With the Talk Test, you have a simple way of monitoring your exercise intensity without the need for gadgets and I have also given you some ideas on how to increase intensity and set goals.

In the last part of the book, I have given you groups of menus. There are sixteen to choose from and they all have recommended warm-ups, top tips and common mistakes. These menus will help you get the most from your Nordic walking whatever your starting point and however you want to use it.

I hope you have found the video coaching links demonstrating the Nordic walking technique a useful accompanying guide. It's often easier to learn something when you see it in action. Finally, do not be disheartened if you don't pick up the technique straight away. Practice really does make perfect when it comes to Nordic walking and if you follow the four golden rules, you will soon have an excellent action and be Nordic walking your way to a fitter, stronger, happier you.

REFERENCES

1. G Stewart, *The Complete Guide to Nordic Walking* (Bloomsbury Sport, 2014)

2. T Rutlin, Exerstrider, www.exerstrider.com (no date), accessed 22 October 2022

3. M Tschentscher, D Niederseer and J Niebauer, 'Health benefits of Nordic walking: A systematic review', *American Journal of Preventive Medicine*, 44 (2013), 76–84, https://doi.org/10.1016/j.amepre.2012.09.043

4. Public Health England, *Muscle and bone strengthening and balance activities for general health benefits in adults and older adults* (2018), https://assets.publishing.service.gov.uk/government/uploads/system/uploads/attachment_data/file/721874/MBSBA_evidence_review.pdf, accessed 22 October 2022

5. N Kakouris, N Yener and D Fong, 'A systematic review of running-related musculoskeletal injuries in runners', *Journal of Sport and Health Science*, 10/5 (2021), 513–522, www.sciencedirect.com/science/article/pii/S2095254621000454#bib0005, accessed 22 October 2022

6. M Hagen, EM Hennig and P Stieldorf, 'Lower and upper extremity loading in nordic walking in comparison with walking and running', *Journal of Applied Biomechanics*, 27/1 (2011), 22–31, doi:10.1123/jab.27.1.22

7. London School of Economics, 'Regular brisk walking is best exercise for keeping weight down' (2015), www.lse.ac.uk/lse-health/news-events/2015/brisk-walking, accessed 6 October 2022

8. V Muollo, AP Rossi, C Milanese et al, 'The effects of exercise and diet program in overweight people – Nordic walking versus walking', *Clinical Interventions in Aging*, 14 (2019), 1555–1565, doi.org/10.2147/CIA.S217570

9. M Tschentscher, D Niederseer and J Niebauer, 'Health benefits of Nordic walking: A systematic review', *American Journal of Preventive Medicine*, 44 (2013), 76–84, https://doi.org/10.1016/j.amepre.2012.09.043

10. Public Health England, *Everybody active, every day: An evidence-based approach* (2014), https://assets.publishing.service.gov.uk/government/uploads/system/uploads/attachment_data/file/374914/Framework_13.pdf, accessed 22 October 2022

11. Mental Health Foundation, 'Nature: How connecting with nature benefits our mental health' (2021), www.mentalhealth.org.uk/our-work/research/nature-how-connecting-nature-benefits-our-mental-health, accessed 22 October 2022

12. NHS, '5 steps to mental wellbeing' (no date), www.nhs.uk/mental-health/self-help/guides-tools-and-activities/five-steps-to-mental-wellbeing, accessed 6 October 2022

13. The Office for Health Improvement and Disparities, 'Physical activity: Applying All Our Health' (GOV.uk, 2022), www.gov.uk/government/publications/physical-activity-applying-all-our-health/physical-activity-applying-all-our-health, accessed 22 October 2022

14. M Tschentscher, D Niederseer and J Niebauer, 'Health benefits of Nordic walking: A systematic review', *American Journal of Preventive Medicine*, 44 (2013), 76–84, https://doi.org/10.1016/j.amepre.2012.09.043

15. DS Silverberg and A Prejserowicz, 'Nordic walking can reduce back, hip and knee pain while walking but is rarely utilized as a form of treatment for these conditions by health professionals', *International Journal of Neurorehabilitation*, 5/2 (2018), http://doi.org/10.4172/2376-0281.1000312

16. R O'Donovan and N Kennedy, "Four legs instead of two" – perspectives on a Nordic walking-based walking programme among people with arthritis', *Disability and Rehabilitation*, 37/18 (2014), 1–8, http://doi.org/10.3109/09638288.2014.972591

17. Chartered Society of Physiotherapy, 'Study finds Nordic walking could help inflammatory rheumatic diseases' (2018), www.csp.org.uk/news/2018-12-11-study-finds-nordic-walking-could-help-inflammatory-rheumatic-diseases, accessed 5 December 2022

18. GC Machado, CG Maher, PH Ferreira et al, 'Non-steroidal anti-inflammatory drugs for spinal pain: A systematic review and meta-analysis', *Annals of the Rheumatic Diseases*, 76/7 (2017), 1269–1278, doi:10.1136/annrheumdis-2016-210597

19. LP Revord, KV Lomond, PV Loubert et al, 'Acute effects of walking with Nordic poles in persons with mild to moderate low-back pain', *International Journal of Exercise Science*, 9/4 (2016), 507–513, www.ncbi.nlm.nih.gov/pmc/articles/PMC5154717, accessed 6 October 2022

20. DS Silverberg and A Prejserowicz, 'Nordic walking can reduce back, hip and knee pain while walking but is rarely utilized as a form of treatment for these conditions by health professionals', *International Journal of Neurorehabilitation*, 5/2 (2018), http://doi.org/10.4172/2376-0281.1000312

21. DS Silverberg and A Prejserowicz, 'Nordic walking can reduce back, hip and knee pain while walking but is rarely utilized as a form of treatment for these conditions by health professionals', *International Journal of Neurorehabilitation*, 5/2 (2018), http://doi.org/10.4172/2376-0281.1000312

22. Birmingham Osteopathy, 'Osteoporosis' (no date), www.birminghamosteopathy.co.uk/osteoporosis-birmingham-osteopath.html, accessed 5 December 2022

23. The Office for Health Improvement and Disparities, 'Physical activity: Applying All Our Health' (GOV.uk, 2022), www.gov.uk/government/publications/physical-activity-applying-all-our-health/physical-activity-applying-all-our-health, accessed 6 October 2022

24. X Du, C Zhang, X Zhang et al, 'The impact of Nordic walking on bone properties in postmenopausal women with pre-diabetes and non-alcohol fatty liver disease', *International Journal of Environmental Research and Public Health*, 18/14 (2021), http://doi.org/10.3390/ijerph18147570

25. T Kato, T Tomioka, T Yamashita et al, 'Nordic walking increases distal radius bone mineral content in young women', *Journal of Sports Science and Medicine*, 19/2 (2020), 237–244, www.ncbi.nlm.nih.gov/pmc/articles/PMC7196759, accessed 6 October 2022

26. British Heart Foundation, *UK Factsheet* (2022), www.bhf.org.uk/-/media/files/research/heart-statistics/bhf-cvd-statistics---uk-factsheet.pdf, accessed 5 December 2022

27. British Heart Foundation, *UK Factsheet* (2022), www.bhf.org.uk/-/media/files/research/heart-statistics/bhf-cvd-statistics---uk-factsheet.pdf, accessed 5 December 2022

28. M Tschentscher, D Niederseer and J Niebauer, 'Health benefits of Nordic walking: A systematic review', *American Journal of Preventive Medicine*, 44 (2013), 76–84, https://doi.org/10.1016/j.amepre.2012.09.043

29. L Cugusi, A Manca, TJ Yeo et al, 'Nordic walking for individuals with cardiovascular disease: A systematic review and meta-analysis of randomized controlled trials', *European Journal of Preventive Cardiology*, 24/18 (2017), 1938–1955, http://doi.org/10.1177/2047487317738592

30. C Spafford, C Oakley and JD Beard, 'Randomized clinical trial comparing nordic pole walking and a standard home exercise programme in patients with intermittent claudication', *The British Journal of Surgery*, 101/7 (2014), 760–7, doi:10.1002/bjs.9519

31. E Kessels, O Husson and CM van der Feltz-Cornelis, 'The effect of exercise on cancer-related fatigue in cancer survivors: A systematic review and meta-analysis', *Neuropsychiatric Disease and Treatment*, 14 (2018), 479–494, www.ncbi.nlm.nih.gov/pmc/articles/PMC5810532, accessed 6 October 2022

32. HY Chiu, HC Huang, PY Chen et al, 'Walking improves sleep in individuals with cancer: A meta-analysis of randomized, controlled trials', *Oncology Nursing Forum*, 42/2 (2015), 54–62, http://doi.org/10.1188/15.ONF.E54-E62

33. MA Sanchez-Lastra, J Torres, I Martinez-Lemos et al, 'Nordic walking for women with breast cancer: A systematic review', *European Journal of Cancer Care*, 28/6 (2019), http://doi.org/10.1111/ecc.13130

34. NHS, 'About dementia' (no date), www.nhs.uk/conditions/dementia/about, accessed 5 December 2022

35. H van Praag, 'Neurogenesis and exercise: Past and future directions', *Neuromolecular Medicine*, 10/2 (2008), 128–40, http://doi.org/10.1007/s12017-008-8028-z

36. Alzheimer's Society, 'Physical exercise and dementia' (no date), www.alzheimers.org.uk/about-dementia/risk-factors-and-prevention/physical-exercise, accessed 6 October 2022

37. The Office for Health Improvement and Disparities, 'Physical activity: Applying All Our Health' (GOV.uk, 2022), www.gov.uk/government/publications/physical-activity-applying-all-our-health/physical-activity-applying-all-our-health, accessed 22 October 2022

38. Parkinson's Foundation, *Fitness Counts: A body guide to Parkinson's Disease* (no date), www.parkinson.org/sites/default/files/Fitness_Counts.pdf, accessed 26 October 2022

39. I Reuter, S Mehnert, P Leone et al, 'Effects of a flexibility and relaxation programme, walking, and Nordic walking on Parkinson's disease', *Journal of Aging Research*, (2011), http://doi.org/10.4061/2011/232473

40. Diabetes UK, 'Diabetes and exercise' (no date), www.diabetes.org.uk/guide-to-diabetes/managing-your-diabetes/exercise, accessed 26 October 2022

41. F Sentinelli, V La Cava, R Serpe et al, 'Positive effects of Nordic walking on anthropometric and metabolic variables in women with type 2 diabetes mellitus', *Science & Sports*, 30/1 (2015), 25–32, http://doi.org/10.1016/j.scispo.2014.10.005

42. KK Hansraj, 'Assessment of stresses in the cervical spine caused by posture and position of the head', *Surgical Technology International*, 25 (2014), 277–9, https://pubmed.ncbi.nlm.nih.gov/25393825, accessed 6 October 2022

43. IA Kapandji, *The Physiology of the Joints Volume 3* (Handspring, 2019)

44. H Zafar, A Albarrati, AH Alghadir et al, 'Effect of different head-neck postures on the respiratory function in healthy males', *BioMed Research International*, (2018), http://doi.org/10.1155/2018/4518269

45. Public Health England, 'Health matters: Getting every adult active every day' (no date), www.gov.uk/government/publications/health-matters-getting-every-adult-active-every-day/health-matters-getting-every-adult-active-every-day, accessed 26 October 2022

46. American Lung Association, 'Lung capacity and aging' (2021), www.lung.org/lung-health-diseases/how-lungs-work/lung-capacity-and-aging, accessed 26 October 2022

47. H Pontzer, JH Holloway, DA Raichlen et al, 'Control and function of arm swing in human walking and running', *Journal of Experimental Biology*, 212/4 (2009), 523–34, http://doi.org/10.1242/jeb.024927

48. P Meyns, SM Bruijn and J Duysens, 'The how and why of arm swing during human walking', *Gait & Posture*, 38/4 (2013), 555–62, http://doi.org/10.1016/j.gaitpost.2013.02.006

49. Department of Health and Social Care, *UK Chief Medical Officers' Physical Activity Guidelines,* (GOV.uk, 2019), https://assets.publishing.service.gov.uk/government/uploads/system/uploads/attachment_data/file/832868/uk-chief-medical-officers-physical-activity-guidelines.pdf, accessed 6 October 2022

50. JL Reed and AL Pipe, 'The talk test: A useful tool for prescribing and monitoring exercise intensity', *Current Opinion in Cardiology,* 29/5 (2014), 475–80, http://doi.org/10.1097/HCO.0000000000000097

51. C Tudor-Locke, H Han, EJ Aguiar et al, 'How fast is fast enough? Walking cadence (steps/min) as a practical estimate of intensity in adults: A narrative review', *British Journal of Sports Medicine*, 52/12 (2017), https://bjsm.bmj.com/content/52/12/776, accessed 6 October 2022

52. M Tschentscher, D Niederseer and J Niebauer, 'Health benefits of Nordic walking: A systematic review', *American Journal of Preventive Medicine*, 44 (2013), 76–84, https://doi.org/10.1016/j.amepre.2012.09.043

53. EA Willis, SA Creasy, JJ Honas et al, 'The effects of exercise session timing on weight loss and components of energy balance: Midwest exercise trial 2', *International Journal of Obesity*, 44 (2020), 114–124, https://doi.org/10.1038/s41366-019-0409-x

54. NHS Rotherham Doncaster and South Humber, *Sweaty Feet: Advice for effective care* (2017), www.rdash.nhs.uk/wp-content/uploads/2014/02/Sweaty-feet-leaflet.pdf, accessed 26 October 2022

55. CG Araujo, CG de Souza e Silva, JA Laukkanen et al, 'Successful 10-second one-legged stance performance predicts survival in middle-aged and older individuals', *British Journal of Sports Medicine*, 56/17 (2021), https://bjsm.bmj.com/content/early/2022/06/22/bjsports-2021-105360, accessed 6 October 2022

56. J Dabrowska, M Dabrowska-Galas, M Rutkowska et al, 'Twelve-week exercise taining and the quality of life in menopausal women – clinical trial', *Menopause Review*, 15/1 (2016), 20–25, http://doi.org/10.5114/pm.2016.58769

57. E Volpi, R Nazemi and S Fujita, 'Muscle tissue changes with aging', *Current Opinion in Clinical Nutrition & Metabolic Care*, 7/4 (2004), 405–410, http://doi.org/10.1097/01.mco.0000134362.76653.b2

58. EJ Howden, S Sarma, JS Lawley et al, 'Reversing the cardiac effects of sedentary aging in middle age – a randomized controlled trial', *Circulation*, 137/15 (2018), 1549–1560, https://doi.org/10.1161/CIRCULATIONAHA.117.030617

59. Department of Health and Social Care, *UK Chief Medical Officers' Physical Activity Guidelines* (GOV.uk, 2019), https://assets.publishing.service.gov.uk/government/uploads/system/uploads/attachment_data/file/832868/uk-chief-medical-officers-physical-activity-guidelines.pdf, accessed 6 October 2022

60. EJ Howden, S Sarma, JS Lawley et al, 'Reversing the cardiac effects of sedentary aging in middle age – a randomized controlled trial', *Circulation*, 137/15 (2018), 1549–1560, https://doi.org/10.1161/CIRCULATIONAHA.117.030617

61. Royal Osteoporosis Society, *Exercise and physical activity for osteoporosis and bone health* (2019), https://theros.org.uk/information-and-support/osteoporosis/living-with-osteoporosis/exercise-and-physical-activity-for-osteoporosis, accessed 6 October 2022

62. Cancer Research, 'What are the benefits of exercise?' (no date), www.cancerresearchuk.org/about-cancer/causes-of-cancer/physical-activity-and-cancer/what-are-the-benefits-of-exercise, accessed 5 December 2022

63. Macmillan Cancer Support, *Physical Activity and Cancer* (2019), https://bit.ly/3SLM2jC, accessed 26 October 2022

64. Parkinson's UK, 'Physical activity and exercise' (no date), www.parkinsons.org.uk/information-and-support/exercise, accessed 6 October 2022

65. Parkinson's UK, 'Physical activity and exercise' (no date), www.parkinsons.org.uk/information-and-support/exercise, accessed 30 October 2022

66. National Institute for Health and Care Excellence, 'Asthma: What is the prevalence of asthma?' (2022), https://cks.nice.org.uk/topics/asthma/background-information/prevalence, accessed 6 October 2022

67. Diabetes UK, 'Diabetes and exercise' (no date), www.diabetes.org.uk/guide-to-diabetes/managing-your-diabetes/exercise, accessed 26 October 2022

68. Diabetes UK, 'Reversing Type 2 diabetes' (no date), www.diabetes.org.uk/diabetes-the-basics/type-2-reverse, accessed 26 October 2022

RESOURCES

Below are some useful resources and links to further information that you may find helpful on your Nordic walking journey.

Where to buy Nordic walking poles

There aren't many outdoor activity shops that have a good selection of Nordic walking poles, so you are best off buying them online. Googling 'buy Nordic walking poles' should bring up lots of options, but two reliable Nordic walking online stores are:

- Nordic Walk Store (www.nordicwalk.store)
- Leki (www.leki.co.uk)

Fitness tracking apps

There are a large number of apps that you can download onto your smartphone and use to record steps, distance, pace, route, calories and elevation, plus get help with goal setting and much more. There are lots to choose from, but three that I like are:

- Strava (www.strava.com)
- MapMyWalk (www.mapmywalk.com)
- Runkeeper (https://runkeeper.com/cms)

Map and walking route apps

You can access Ordnance Survey maps, find walking routes and challenges, record routes and much more using map and walking route apps. Here are three I enjoy using:

- OS Maps (https://shop.ordnancesurvey.co.uk/apps)
- Outdooractive (www.outdooractive.com)
- Go Jauntly (www.gojauntly.com)

Wildlife apps

If you want to identify wildflowers, trees and other wildlife that you spot while on the go, you can now use apps instead of carrying books. Three of the best are:

- iNaturalist (www.inaturalist.org)
- PictureThis (www.picturethisai.com)
- Woodland Trust (tree identifier) (www.woodlandtrust.org.uk/trees-woods-and-wildlife/british-trees/tree-id-app)

Walking holidays

There are many companies offering walking holidays, in groups, guided or self-guided. Three that I would particularly recommend are:

- Self-guided, Inntravel (www.inntravel.co.uk/walking-holidays)
- Guided, Exodus (www.exodus.co.uk/activities/walking-holidays)
- Bespoke, Shearwater Travel (www.shearwatertravel.co.uk)

ACKNOWLEDGEMENTS

Writing this book would not have been possible without the inspiration, help, and support of some special people.

My husband Adrian, for his wisdom, humour and patience and our children Chris, Matt and Sammy, who have had no option but to live and breathe my passion for Nordic walking for the majority of their lives. Thank you.

To the wonderful Bristol Nordic walkers for the happy years of walking together; to the walkers who have allowed me to feature them in this book; and to everyone else who has Nordic walked with me along the way.

Thank you to everyone who has given their support, encouragement, and feedback so generously, particularly Nicola Boyce, Helen Milne, Mark Ware, Faith Davey, Jane Shearer, Katharine Green, Clare Long, Polly Bingley, Jenny Fennell, Liz Carver, Beth Fallon, Sally Norton and my Book Writing Team.

Thank you, too, to my expert contributors, Naomi Green, Footworks Bristol, www.footworksbristol.com/naomi-green.html and Minia Alonso, Bristol Massage Clinic, https://bristolmassageclinic.co.uk

To the amazing Lucy McCarraher and my fellow authors in the book mentoring and mastermind writing group for their unswerving belief and support; to my wonderful illustrator Rachel Hall; and to my publishers Rethink Press, especially Abi Willford, Helen Lanz, Sarah Marchant, and Anke Ueberberg.

Finally, to the memory of Annie Briggs who kickstarted my Nordic walking career and who I know is still much missed by all those in Norfolk.

THE AUTHOR

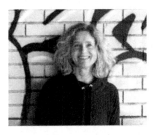 Vicky Welsh is one of England's most experienced Nordic walking instructors and has been teaching Nordic walking for over twelve years. She is a National Trainer for the International Nordic Walking Federation (INWA), has written extensively about Nordic walking and has spoken regularly on local and national radio about Nordic walking, health and fitness.

Vicky has taught hundreds of people of all fitness levels to Nordic walk and has used her extensive knowledge as a qualified personal fitness trainer to develop bespoke Nordic walking programmes. She has strong links with local fitness and health professionals and regularly consults with them to bring new ideas to her Nordic walking.

In 2010, Vicky founded an award-winning Nordic walking business in her hometown of Bristol, growing it into one of the largest Nordic walking clubs in the country. She created a range of Nordic walking classes to suit all fitness levels and introduced scenic walks, weekends away and club challenges, writing training schedules, giving tips and advice and providing support and encouragement.

Vicky offers weekend Nordic walking courses and tailored Nordic walking workshops in Bristol. She is also helping to develop free and low-cost Nordic walking courses and classes across South West England. Vicky herself Nordic walks every day, usually accompanied by her springer spaniel, Alfie.

You can contact Vicky on:
- 🌐 www.letswalknordic.com
- ✉ vicky@letswalknordic.com
- 📘 Letswalknordic
- 📷 Letswalknordic

Printed in Great Britain
by Amazon

18135362R00108